It's Personal
HIV/AIDS Real stories about Real People

The Day the Ground Fell from Under Me

by

Mary S. Jones

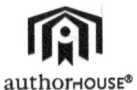

authorHOUSE®

AuthorHouse™
1663 Liberty Drive, Suite 200
Bloomington, IN 47403
www.authorhouse.com
Phone: 1-800-839-8640

First published by AuthorHouse 3/26/2008

ISBN: 978-1-4343-5416-7 (sc)

Library of Congress Control Number: 2008902369

Printed in the United States of America
Bloomington, Indiana

This book is printed on acid-free paper.

Contents

ACKNOWLEDGMENTS

To sit down and write anything can be a challenge; facing a blank page and trying to find the first letter or word can cause all kinds of emotions to become stirred within your spirit. I never considered myself a writer, but the stories and encouragement of others have helped me put my life and dreams on paper. The stories contained herein, which were shared with me, are reflections of life with pitfalls, potholes, and detours, but they're mostly a determination to live. I would like to personally thank each of you for enriching, enhancing, and changing my life forever. I now live each day with a part of your world within me, and I wouldn't want anything to change that. I love you and will forever honor your honesty in telling me, and the world, your stories.

I am indebted to a host of individual who have helped and watch me grow over the past years. Thanks to Delois Bolden who took me under her wing and allowed me to soar to greater heights. To Dr. Jobese Okwumabua, my advisor and mentor, but mostly my friend; your encouragement and support can never be expressed in words.

To all my friends at Friends for Life, Inc., thank you. To Bishop Isaac Akorli (Grace, Bernice, Wisdom, Princilla) and extended family; thanks for opening your home and sharing your world. (Ghana, West Africa). To Pastor Kenneth T. Whalum, Jr., and Shelia, I love you, and would not be on this endless journey without your wonderful teachings and examples. You have truly transformed my life and dreams. To the rest of my New Olivet Baptist Church family, I love you, too. I would like to thank my mother, Roberta Scott, my father, Johnny Scott, my sisters, Jo Ann and Tonya, and my brothers, Johnny, Robin, and Darren. Growing up with ya'll was fantastic! To my many nieces, nephews, cousins, aunts, and uncles, thanks. Phillip and Hannah, the sky is your limit; shoot for it. I want to say thanks to my extended family; Cheryl, Fred, Maurice, Deushawn, and all the aunts, uncles, nieces, nephews and cousins. Shirley and Sharon, thanks for the late night read.

To my son, William, I love you and I continue to trust God to do what he promised. Thanks for my grandsons. My greatest thanks go to Dwayne thank you for allowing God to use you. Your encouragement and support have been one of my greatest assets. Thanks for adding that much-needed spark to my dreams. I love you. To you the reader, thank you.

PREFACE

It is difficult if not impossible to overlook the fact that HIV/AIDS is real and life changing. This disease has shown devastation in every community, city, state, nation, and even our world. This disease does not discriminate and neither does it show respect for dreams to come. We, as people, did not take notice of the warning that was revealed to us over twenty-seven years ago, and now we must suffer the consequences of lives altered.

Although medical science has made wonderful breakthroughs in research and medicine, more is needed. Recent advances in medication regimens for the treatment of HIV/AIDS have been responsible not only for reducing the AIDS death rate, but also for extending the trajectory from diagnosis, to AIDS symptoms, and to death. For some patients, the new medications are not easy to take. Drug regimens are often complicated, and side effects are common and unpleasant. For many, adherence failure leads to drug resistance and limited treatment options. We must still ensure that AIDS drugs are both affordable and accessible for all who need them.

Young people have been the hardest hit by this pandemic. Since symptoms of HIV infection may take ten or more years to manifest themselves, diagnoses of AIDS in twenty-year-olds may be an indicator of infection during their teen years.

As is true in most regions of the United States, HIV and AIDS disproportionately affect African Americans, females, and heterosexuals. The rate among women continues to rise. Men who have sex with men comprise their greatest risk factor, while heterosexual sex also contributes to a great portion of new infections. Although the numbers are disproportionately represented, no race or nationality has been excluded. This virus has claimed the lives of Whites, Latinos, Asian-Americans and Native Americans.

Stopping the spread of HIV/AIDS has many components. We need to increase education and funds, provide training and twenty-four-hour access to information, service and treatment; and encourage the FDA to speed the approval process for other less expensive drugs. HIV/AIDS health care and services are inadequate and are frequently delivered in a fragmented manner. Gaps in these services need to be developed into a more comprehensive and coordinated system. By suggesting that we have a lot of work ahead of us, I am not implying that we have not crossed and conquered many milestones. The fight is not over.

The fight does not end in the United States. We must include the lives of others. My trip to Ghana, West Africa was life changing. Imagine in the year 2007 living without running water, electricity, a home, or access to basic medical care. I experienced it first hand. Although we spoke different languages, through an interrupter I was able to feel and share their desire for help. Basic information about HIV/AIDS was something many had never heard. Think about it; something in your community that is taking the lives of those around you and you don't know how to protect yourself. The greatest issue facing them is the same one we face—lack of education and economics. I've begun to do my part through education and opening The Grace and Mary Vocational Training School. Students are taught the skills of sewing and tailoring to better their lives. Let me stop here to thank each of you who helped make that possible through your donations and support. I will forever be grateful to you.

Allow me now to introduce a suggestion that this disease has become "Personal." The evidence lies in the pages of this book. The people and lives that have been touched by this virus are real. As an educator and service provider for over fifteen years, I have seen its affect on lives and families. To stand face to face with someone and tell them that this virus does not discriminate, and then to see that same individual less than two years later for service because they are infected is sometimes a hard pill to swallow. No one whom I know has intentionally gotten infected. We still want to believe that it is the drug users, uneducated, lower social economic status, or the neighborhood that causes one to get infected. None of these are absolute truths. It is not who you are, but what you do, that puts you at risk for this virus. This virus is sexually transmitted; if you have sex with someone who is infected, you can contract this virus.

What is so amazing is that the majority of infected people don't look like they are infected. But I must ask, what does an infected individual look like? There are no specific characteristics. The only way to know if you or your partner is infected is to be tested. Ladies, it is time to talk to your girlfriends. Men, it is time to talk to your boys. Pastors, it is time to talk to your congregations. Doctors, it is time to talk to your patients, and parents, it is time to talk to your children. It's no longer business. It's personal.

INTRODUCTION

It still remains true that a picture is worth a thousand words. If we took a snapshot of HIV/AIDS today, and looked at the picture two years from now, it would only capture that moment in time and nothing else. The faces and lives of individuals continuously change. They reflect different moments of when the ground fell from under them. To hear that someone died from complications of AIDS is still unheard of even today, even after more than twenty-five years of its existence. I dare we disrespect the dead by identifying it as the cause of death on their obituary—never knowing whether it could save someone's life right there in the church.

The shame and stigma associated with this virus has paralyzed a nation and sent it into silence. If we continue to ignore the elephant in the middle of our living room, it doesn't mean that the elephant does not exist, and neither will it go away. We fuel the spread of HIV/AIDS to a certain degree by simply ignoring it. This causes concerned parents to send their children out into the real world with feel-good thoughts but no real protection.

Take notice of this picture perfect family, who, in their minds, think they have prepared their child for the world on the other side of their doors. How many of us would agree that if asked the right question, by the right person, and at the right time, we might change our thoughts to what we know to be true. The virus is found in blood, semen, vaginal fluids, and in some cases, breast milk. It is transmitted through vaginal, anal, and oral sex. Having unprotected sex with an infected individual puts you at risk for the virus.

Casual contact is not our enemy when it comes to this virus. If that had ever been the case, we would all be infected. You cannot look at someone and assume they have the virus. Through years of research and medical advancement, we are now able to treat individuals to a point where they may live long and productive lives. This does not give you the green light to live life as you choose. The questions about past sex partners need to be asked of anyone you have sexual contact with.

Why not get tested together? Not knowing is not safe. The virus has a window period where it cannot be detected by the test. The window period is up to three months after being infected. Therefore, it is important that after your first test for HIV, that you are careful what you do and return for the follow-up test. It amazes me when people say they get tested all the time. I'm always wondering, why? I think I know the answer. We know what we are doing, and we know that HIV does not discriminate. Yet, we don't want to give up certain behaviors or habits. I say to you, it is time to give up the old habits to save your life. Stop playing Russian roulette.

Once infected with HIV, there is no going back. There is no changing your mind. There is no second chance, and there is no cure.

THIS IS ASHLEY'S STORY

After five years of marriage, Angela and Daniel tried every means available to them to have a child. After two years, they gave up all hope. Six months later, Angela was pregnant. They didn't care if the child was a boy or a girl. They just wanted to have a healthy child. Nine months later, Ashley was born healthy, bright eyed and very active. Ashley was her parents' pride and joy. Angela and Daniel made a vow to raise their daughter in a Christian household and they did.

Angela was an accountant and Daniel worked in pharmaceutical sales. They lived in the suburbs, took family vacations, and started a college fund for Ashley when she was only six months old. Life was good. Ashley sailed through childhood and her teen years with no problems. She was an honor student, and never gave her parents any trouble. Her extra curriculum activities included soccer, basketball, dancing, singing in the youth choir at their church, volunteering to feed the homeless during the holiday seasons, and visiting senior citizens of their church. Ashley was the perfect child and her life's dream was to become a lawyer.

Academics paid off for Ashley. She was given a full scholarship to attend the University of Mississippi in Oxford, Mississippi. Ashley achieved academic excellence during her freshman and sophomore years with a 4.0 GPA. Her parents were very proud. They used a portion of her school funds to purchase a car for her, and they rented an apartment for her.

Ashley was very active in the pre-law club and she was co-captain of the debate team, which required some travel. She competed within the region, Hawaii, and Washington, DC where she excelled well above her peers. Ashley was slowly becoming the school's prized competitor. Mr. Terrance Lemon was the team's sponsor.

Terrance was from California. He was an only child and would be the fourth generation of lawyers in his family. He was very handsome and well-groomed. His hazel eyes were an added bonus to his chestnut skin tone. Standing six-feet tall, he always walked as if he had a rod in his back—military style with a commanding disposition. He was very friendly and dedicated to his studies. Terrance lived with his homeboy, Lance. As a fourth-year law student, he took a strong liking and interest in Ashley's talents. He became her coach and mentor. They spent some evenings together and he would coach her on different debating skills. Mr. Lemon insisted that Ashley call him Terrance.

Ashley was in awe of Terrance's attention. She began to have feelings beyond just coach/mentor for Terrance. Terrance also felt something special for Ashley. She was now twenty years old and Terrance was six years her senior. However, Ashley didn't care. She began to make extra efforts for his attention and he went along with the plan.

Ashley's mind continuously flashed back to her upbringing when she thought about being intimate with Terrance. She had been encouraged to save her virginity until marriage, but her desire for Terrance was very strong. Desire would override her vow of virginity. Ashley heard that Terrance would be leaving at the end of the year, so she decided to make her move.

Terrance called Ashley with some exciting news. He told her that she had been invited to participate in a national debate competition in the spring, she had only a week to respond to the invitation. Excited, Ashley knew this would be the perfect time for her to make her feelings known. She asked Terrance if he would bring the papers to her apartment. He agreed. Her plan was now in motion. Ashley went about setting the mood.

Ashley lit candles in the living room, fluffed the pillows on the sofa, threw some chocolate chip cookies in the oven, chilled a bottle of wine, opened her laptop on the kitchen table, showered, and covered every inch of her body with Victoria's Secret Amber Romance body lotion and spray. She pulled her hair up in a ponytail and waited for Terrance to arrive. The doorbell rang right on schedule at 7:30 p.m.,

"Come in, Terrance."

Terrance entered the apartment and immediately commented on the smell of fresh cookies that filled the room. He handed Ashley an envelope. Ashley offered him a cookie as he followed her to the kitchen. She read the invitation and asked Terrance if he thought she should accept. Terrance told her with the biggest smile, not only should she accept, he told her she would win. Ashley smiled as she checked the "Will participate" box on the invitation. Then she sealed the invite, in preparation for mailing it.

"This calls for a celebration," Ashley said, as she opened the refrigerator.

She brought out a bottle of White Zinfandel.

Passing the bottle to Terrance, she asked, "Will you do the honors?"

Hours later, Terrance kissed Ashley on her forehead before he rolled out of her bed. He thanked her for a wonderful and memorable evening, but insisted that he must get home before Lance put out an APB on him. Ashley grabbed her robe and walked Terrance to the door. They kissed and Terrance promised to drop

Ashley's response in the mail on his way home. Ashley blew out the candles on her way to the bedroom, then stopped to look at herself in the mirror. Yesterday a girl, today a woman—thanks, Terrance. She smiled as she walked away.

Terrance looked for Ashley the next day on campus and she was nowhere to be found. She had missed all her classes, which was something very out of character for her. He called her apartment to check on her. She answered the phone in a very weak voice.

Terrance asked, "Are you okay?"

"Yes," she replied, "just the sniffles or something. I'll be fine."

He offered to bring over some juice.

She replied, "No, thanks, I don't want you to catch whatever it is I have."

"Okay," he said, "I'll check on you later. Get some rest."

Then he hung up the phone.

Ashley was out of it for about three days. When she finally felt better, she and Terrance met for lunch. As Ashley prepared for mid-term exams and Thanksgiving break, she and Terrance had a rendezvous five more times at her place. They became closer, and he told her of his dreams and hopes for the future. She, in return, told him of her dreams of one day being the most recognizable lawyer for defending abused women. She also spoke of being married and having children—two boys and a girl. Terrance told her she could have anything she put her mind to. Their time together became precious in Ashley's world.

Ashley was always careful when she and Terrance had sex, but there were a couple of times when the condoms burst and Ashley didn't have time in her schedule for any unwanted pregnancy, so she decided to make a doctor's appointment to get birth control pills.

At Ashley's appointment, the doctor suggested she be tested for HIV. She told her there was nothing to worry about apart from her routine checkup. Ashley received a sample of birth control pills and a prescription for six months of refills. Midterms were over and Ashley was headed home for the holidays. She and Terrance would not see each other for a few days, so one for the road was in order.

Thanksgiving at home with family and friends was great. Ashley told her family about her invitation to participate in the national debate competition. Everyone was so excited and they promised to be there to cheer her on. When the weekend was over, Ashley hit the road before dark. She kissed her parents good-bye and headed up the highway to her place.

She stopped at her mailbox to gather her mail before going to her apartment. Collapsing on the sofa, she began to thumb through all the after-Thanksgiving sales and free credit cards offers. She noticed the light flashing on her answering machine. Hoping there was a message from Terrance, she hit the play button.

The recording said, "Ashley, this is Dr. Young. Please give us a call at the office when you get this message."

The next message was from Terrance, saying that he would not be returning to town as planned. Lance had gotten sick over the holidays and was in the hospital. He promised to call her later. Ashley was disappointed and continued thumbing through her mail. On the floor, she noticed a white envelope which had fallen out of the pile. She picked it up and saw that it is from the local health department, stamped confidential. She ripped the letter open, and read the message.

YOUR NAME HAS BEEN REPORTED TO OUR AGENCY AS HAVING HIV ANTIBODIES IN

YOUR BLOOD. PLEASE CONTACT US AS SOON
AS POSSIBLE FOR SCREENING.

THANKS,

What would Ashley do now with her hopes and dreams? Would
she tell Terrance, her parents, or her friends?

Ashley is not real, and neither is her story. However, this has
become a scene all around the world with more than twenty-five
million people having died of AIDS, and forty million currently
infected with HIV. Today, more than one million Americans
are HIV positive—more women, more African-Americans, and
more heterosexuals. At first, it was just something we read in the
newspapers, magazines, or in school textbooks. Now, the disease
has a personal face as we lose people we know and love.

This has been the case for me over the past fifteen years. I have
lost relatives, loved ones, and friends to a disease that takes the lives
of people too young, too fast, and too many. These are individuals
I loved, but for whatever reason have been forgotten and erased
from society.

In an effort to preserve the memories of real people, I've decided,
with their approval, to tell their stories. Although infected, they
deserve to be remembered by society for their time here.

In the pages of this book, I hope you can feel the pulse of life
as individuals tell stories of their past, present and future. Some of
the names have been changed to protect their privacy, while others
wanted the world to know them as real people who are living with
a real disease.

Please do not take this as an opportunity to exclude yourself
from this disease. Maybe you graduated from high school, and you
didn't have sex until you thought you were "grown." You never lied

about your age to get an older man or woman. You didn't grow up in the "ghetto." Your best friend told you everything. You don't sleep with those kinds of people. All your friends make seven figure incomes, and live in fabulous homes, drive expensive cars, and you always use protection. Don't forget the time when the heat of the moment took over you judgment; when things happened so fast you convinced yourself that just thos one time... Or the times you got comfortable in your "long-term committed relationship;" off came the protection. Later, you found out your partner was not so committed.

It's personal.
Enjoy!

LOST FRIENDSHIP

SEPTEMBER 15, 1997

As Shelia sat in the small Baptist church, her mother and husband tried to convince her to stand up and look at Candice's body. She had so many emotions bottled up inside, it was impossible to move. The only thing she knew was that her best friend was gone.

Shelia tells the story about her friend's life and their times together with many regrets and heartfelt emotions. Shelia said she was trying to understand what happened. What illness or disease could come into her life and destroy it like this one had done? Did this illness have some secrets inside itself? Its web entangled her into a new world that was not common or familiar. It was like a door that was open, and no matter how hard she tried, she could not close it. I invite you to listen as Shelia describes her life and times with Candice.

Why didn't Candice tell me that she was sick? Didn't she trust me with her innermost secrets? Did she think that I couldn't handle it, or did she think it would change our friendship? Hindsight is 20/20 they say. I wish Candice had trusted me enough to let me try. As days went by, I began to ponder some piercing questions that haunted my days and uneasy nights.

Shelia smiled as she gathered her thoughts about her best friend, and the way their lives had become intertwined in this wonderful journey. Candice and Shelia became friends by accident. They really didn't like each other that much at first, but Shelia always felt like part of their family, due to the closeness that she had with Candice's grandmother. Mrs. Walker was Shelia's Sunday school teacher for many years. Candice's sister, Monica, was good friends with Shelia and they attended community college together. Candice was considered an outsider—an oddball. Candice didn't conform to society like people thought she should. Candice had a child at an early age, and was she was surrounded by questionable influences. Her self-esteem was not the best in the world. She always saw the glass half-empty. Nothing she saw seemed good, so that's how she viewed her life and the world around her. Monica and I were total opposites. Monica was full of young life and wanted to enter into adulthood with great possibility.

Suddenly things and times changed. Monica decided to move to California to live with her mother. Shelia was losing her best friend but she didn't realize she was gaining a new sister who would change her views on life forever.

Candice and Shelia became friends. They were some of the original "Ghetto- Fabulous Girls." They began to date some neighbor guys—boys in the HOOD. Candice started too really like a young man named Mark. On the exterior, Mark seemed to be a cool dude and they had several things in common. They both had sons around the same age, and both children were developmentally challenged with different behaviors. Mark and Candice were inseparable but in a weird way. They became too inseparable. Mark moved in with Candice and her grandparents. Candice would talk about how Mark was becoming hostile with her grandparents; mostly her grandfather. Newly in love, Candice was confused as to where her loyalty should lay. She was confusing love with lust, and violence with caring. Candice thought that love was supposed to be complex, in some strange way. Candice and Mark stayed together for several years.

Monica had settled in California. She and Shelia talked often. Monica was back in town briefly after her grandmother suffered a stroke. Shelia had always kept her informed via phone after she returned to California. They talked about life, love issues, and why they felt confused about so many things at this stage in their lives.

Candice grew tired of the battle between her grandfather and Mark. She wanted to be free of them both. She decided to go out into the world with her son and left them both behind. She got her own place, and began to see life differently—an upswing from years passed. Her relationship with her grandfather was better due to the distance between them. Her son was doing well in school. She was a loyal volunteer at her son's school and her church. After awhile, Candice began to miss the familiar and decided to visit old places to get reacquainted with several of her old friends. She crossed paths with Mark again. Her situation had changed but Mark's character had not. It still amazes me how things change but people's mindsets sometimes stay the same.

Mark and Candice got back together again in their enchanted cottage—her place. Everything appeared to be good for awhile. They were in love/lust again. Several weeks passed and Mark wanted his space. He decided to start spending his weeks elsewhere, but spent the weekends with Candice. She heard he was living with another woman, but Mark convinced her that he was back home with his mother. Things got better between the two of them. Mark began to spend all his time with Candice again.

Neighborhood rumors reached Candice's doorstep. A woman in the neighborhood had died of AIDS and she was one of Mark's lovers. Candice refused to believe that Mark could have had anything to do with someone of this nature. Candice called Shelia and told her the rumor. Candice felt that people were telling lies about Mark, and they wanted to scare her so she wouldn't see him. Candice believed all the gossip was a lie, until the day Mark had to clear his conscious.

Mark told Candice he had something serious to tell her. She wondered what it could be. Did it have anything to do with the rumors that were in the old neighborhood about that woman who died with AIDS? Was he just messing with her? She knew that Mark did a little crack, but she loved him and could help him through that. It didn't matter that he had stolen and sold all her tangible items in the house—TVs, lamps, stereos, telephones, and anything that wasn't bolted down. Mark was about to confess.

Mark began the conversation by saying, "You know I love you, Candice, and I want us to be together forever, but I need to tell you that I'm HIV positive. A friend that I used to kick it with has DIED."

For some of us, the story would end right there, but it didn't.

Candice was very understanding of Mark's situation and called their on-and-off relationship done. Mark moved out. Candice began to focus on herself and her child, but that didn't last long. Familiarity showed its head again. Mark was back. She loved him so much that she would honestly love him to death.

Shelia was shocked when Candice told her that Mark was back in her life. She tried to help Candice remember that Mark had done everything under the sun to her, and now he is HIV positive.

Sheila told her, "Don't put your life on the line for a man who cares nothing about you."

Candice was convinced that Mark loved her, and needed her now more than ever.

Shelia talked to Candice on a regular basis, mostly about Mark. Several months passed since Shelia had actually seen Candice. Shelia was now married and building a future with her husband. Shelia called Candice's grandparent's house looking for her when she couldn't reach her at home. Candice's grandfather said that she was sick and would be coming back to live with him. He invited Shelia to come and visit with them. Shelia had not seen them in awhile, so she stopped by a few days later.

Candice was there. She appeared a little thin, but said she was on a diet. They all chatted about life and the things they were doing. Yeah, they talked a little about Mark. As Shelia chatted with Candice, she became convinced that dieting was not the reason for Candice's weight loss. Shelia left after about an hour but promised them both she would be back to visit.

A few weeks passed. Shelia had talked with Candice and her grandfather but had only visited once. Candice was not looking her best. One night Candice called Shelia and said she needed to go to the emergency room. She wasn't feeling well. Shelia told her she would be right over but she would have to drop her off because she was going to night service at her church. Shelia never knew that this night would be a kingdom lesson that would last forever.

Shelia pulled up to the house to pick Candice up. Candice looked very fragile as she got in the car. They did very little talking during the drive, but Shelia felt a need to drive quickly. Shelia pulled up to the emergency room to drop Candice off.

However, before she could put the car in drive, Candice said in a helpless voice, "Can you stay with me?"

Shelia's heart was broken. The thought of leaving her friend alone in this condition at the hospital was crushing.

She told her, "Yes, I will stay with you."

Candice was immediately placed in an exam room and asked to put on a hospital gown. Shelia helped her onto the exam table and pulled the sheet around her shoulders. She held her hand until the doctor entered the room. He asked Candice numerous questions about her health concerns and several questions about sexual experiences. He lifted the white sheet for a closer look but quickly lowered it, as if he already knew the diagnosis. They ran several tests on Candice and then sent her home.

Several days later, Shelia learned what those tests and symptoms meant—T-cells, viral loads, the lesions, night sweats, and memory loss. They were the signs and symptoms of HIV/AIDS. Candice never told Shelia anything else about her hospital visit and Shelia never asked her. Shelia never knew if Candice told anyone. Shelia believed in her heart that Candice wanted to tell her and maybe she did in her own way.

Shelia called to check on Candice often, but the conversation would always include Mark—how and what he was doing and how concerned Candice was about him. Candice's love for this man was amazing. What kind of love is it that makes you forget about yourself and place your whole being in someone else's hands? Shelia asked Candice questions about whether she was still sleeping with Mark. Her answers were always vague and redirected to another conversation. Shelia felt helpless in her struggle to free or save her friend. Months would pass before Shelia would see her friend. Shelia heard one Sunday that Candice was back in the hospital again.

Shelia was starting a new job on that Monday in September and made plans to visit Candice that Sunday evening. The evening was cloudy and rainy. Shelia's husband tried to get her to wait until Monday after work to visit Candice, but something inside of Shelia gave her an urgency to visit Candice on that day. Shelia and her husband headed to the hospital.

As they entered a hallway inside the hospital, they saw Candice's son and grandfather. Shelia rushed to them. As she entered Candice's room, what she saw hurt her innermost soul. Her heart broke into a million pieces. Her best girlfriend and sister was really sick. Shelia tried to keep from crying. Tears filled her eyes and hurt clutched her heart as she locked eyes with the shell of a woman who was her friend.

The only words her locked vocal chords would release were, "I love you, Candice."

Candice slowly moved her lips to say, "I love you, too."

Their eyes met for the last time as sisters. The two girls who had become women together were now splitting up. Candice died the next day.

Candice's funeral was beautiful. Her white casket was covered with white roses and sprays of greenery were everywhere. The tulips, carnations, forget-me-nots and lilies were in perfect bloom, but church tradition overshadowed the service. Mark was not in attendance due to rumors that a young lady he had been intimate with had learned of his disease and was going to kill him if he showed up. Candice's grandfather and son sat in the front row with tears streaming down their cheeks, and a look of dismay on their faces. The service was officiated by Mark's uncle who was the church pastor.

Many of Candice's friends made their way to the front of the church to view her body. They knew Mark was dying of AIDS and suspected this was the cause of Candice's death. Shelia just watched as everyone looked in the coffin at her friend who had died too soon. Few people expressed their condolences during the service and then Mark's uncle took his position at the podium. He immediately went into character and the traditional Baptist preacher hoop. He began to spout out words that described a young lady who was not Candice. His words echoed throughout the church but were not pleasing to Candice's grandfather. He rose from his front row seat and walked out of the church under a tear-stained face.

On September 15, 1997, as Shelia sat in that church with her heart breaking, she knew now that her girlfriend was free. Her mother and husband tried to convince Shelia to stand up and look at Candice's body. She had so many emotions bottled up inside that it was impossible for her to move. As she cried, her tears also freed her, and she learned her greatest lesson. Self-love is the greatest love of all.

Young but Not So Innocent

November 22, 2006

I couldn't say one word. It felt like the ground had disappeared and I was being sucked into this endless black hole.

Just recovering from a bout of shingles, I sat down to speak with Kay P. I must say the girl looked good. She had a short haircut that framed her face and even wearing her baby blue scrubs gave the impression that she was well put together. Kay P. was your typical young lady growing up in urban America. She had big dreams and high hopes of being a hairstylist to the stars, but something got in the way of those dreams. As her teen years brought about new interest and life-changing consequences, Kay's story is typical; however, viewed by society as just the change of times. She began by explaining how it all started for her.

Kay cleared her throat and said, "I became a teenager, thought I had all the answers, and I couldn't be told anything. I had built a reputation in my neighborhood and school when I failed the seventh and eighth grades for fighting. Now, eighteen years old and in the tenth grade, I'm willing and ready to do whatever to protect my reputation. I was suspended for 180 days for fighting again. It was not my fault. This girl disrespected me and I had to show her that, 'thangs ain't like that; he was my man and I was in love with him. (Kay would fall in love at least four more times before she celebrated her twenty-fourth birthday).

I knew that with a suspension of this kind, there was no way I was going to pass to the next grade. Unable to attend any other school in the system, I decided to drop out. Now I had all the time I needed to hang out, party, drink, or whatever. The relationship between Bob and me didn't last but my best friend didn't let me wallow in my pity. She introduced me to her god-brother. He lived out of state.

We had a long distance relationship. He lived in Indiana. Four months into the phone calls, I knew I was in love. I had never seen this man before but when he suggested that I move in with him, I was more than ready. I was twenty-one, and I could do whatever I wanted to do. My friend and I packed and he came to get us on September 26, 2005. Off we went to celebrate our new lives and my new love. We'll call him, Mr. Telephone Lover.

The living arrangements were cool. My friend and I shared the extra bedroom and Mr. Telephone Lover had his room. As we talked and learned more about each other, things got a little more personal, and the living arrangement changed. In October 2005, I moved into his bedroom. Everything was fun and exciting but the bills still had to be paid. He was on disability. He was deaf in one ear and legally blind in one eye; something I found out after I moved to Indiana. My girlfriend and I were responsible for the electric bill, cable, and food. I got a job during the day at a local bakery, and at night, I worked at Mickey Dee's—you know, McDonalds. Everything was fine.

One day as I was coming home from work, one of our friends from the apartment met me coming up the sidewalk.

"What's up, Jay?"

He was my homeboy, and lived a few doors down in the apartment complex. We had hit it off because we had things in common. We could talk about home, places we hung out, people we knew, and other simple things.

Jay said, "Don't go into that apartment, Kay."

I said, "Boy, what are you talking about?"

He appeared to be a little under the juice, you know, drunk.

He said, "Don't go in that apartment. They are going to hurt you."

I waved him off and kept walking towards the apartment. Shit, I was tired and needed a shower. When I turned the key and entered the apartment, Mr. Telephone Lover and five of his friends were situated all around the living room playing the Play Station 2. I spoke as I walked past them and headed for the bedroom. As I began to prepare to take my shower, a strange feeling came over me, so I decided to wait. Mr. Telephone Lover came into the room and insisted that I take my shower and relax. I loved him, so I wanted to please him.

There were two doors between his friends and me so I decided to take my shower. I could hear them talking in the other room. After getting into the shower, I realized I had forgotten my towel. I got out of the shower, went to the linen closet, and wrapped a towel around me. When I returned to the bathroom, all six men were waiting for me. They tied me up, raped me, burned me with cigarettes, and left me on the floor, balled up in the corner by the commode. My world stopped. I could not believe or understand why someone who said he loved me, had moved me into his home and bed, would do this to me. I crawled to our bedroom, found a pair of shorts and T-shirt, dressed myself, and called the police. I filed a report and then was transported to the hospital. After the examination, it was clear that I needed further treatment. I could not go back to the apartment, so I called my girlfriend (you know, the one who introduced us), told and I told her what had happened.

She said, "Good for you."

I was shattered right there on my phone, I could not believe what I had just heard. Shamed, hurt, embarrassed, alone, and empty, I had to make a choice.

The next morning I woke up in a psychiatric ward in Harvey, Illinois. I spent the next two months trying to put my life back together and get up enough courage to call my mother. I did. On December 15, with the help of a Christian center splitting the eighty-dollar bus fare, I was headed home.

The place I had left only a few months ago had now become my personal prison. I felt ashamed, hurt, and confused. I had lost over fifteen pounds, felt stressed out, and couldn't eat. The Christmas spirit was all around me but it didn't matter. Christmas came and went and I felt the New Year was just time passing on the calendar.

Spring sprung in me and I was ready to live life again. I began to get out and met my new love, Marques. After only five days of talking, I moved in with him and his mother on May 25. By June, his jealousy began to show. He abused me both emotionally and physically. I moved back home with my mother. I still loved him and allowed two weeks of his pleading and apologizing to change my mind. I went back to him—me and my dog. To help curb his jealousy, I didn't work or leave the house unnecessarily.

He was in a car wreck on June 30, and lost his job. The beating became an everyday thing. I can ask myself now why I stayed. All I can say is that I stayed for five months, and it was like living in my new prison. In October, he had new plans that I was not aware of, and he put me and my dog out. Three weeks later, I was back.

Less than a week later, on November 4, after his sister's birthday party, I saw his plan. I walked in the house and there he was with his baby's momma having sex right there in front of me. I said nothing, packed my things, and went back to my mother's house. I sat around for a month, making promises to myself.

On November 13, I was awakened in the middle of the night with a toothache that so painful that breathing was difficult. Walking only made it worse. I applied Orajel and came very close to overdosing on Tylenol. By 6:00 a.m., I was sitting in the emergency room of a local hospital. I sat there for more than eight hours waiting to see a doctor. I could not talk. My tongue and face were swollen. I communicated by writing. The nurse finally called my name, and I was told that I needed to have two teeth extracted. I went into surgery on November 14, and woke up one week later (November 21) in ICU. My mother, sister, brother, and the man who threw me out a month earlier were there. I couldn't talk because of the tubes in my neck, and I had lost the use of my arms and leg. I was moved to a regular room in the hospital. I never will forget that room—3236 E. Wing. My family spent the evening trying to explain what had happened to me.

On November 22, 2006, my doctor made his morning rounds. He walked in, introduced himself, and began explaining that he was going to remove the tubes from my neck, and that I would need physical therapy. The next words out of his mouth were that I had Pumoscystic Carini Puenoumia (PCP) and that I was HIV positive. Right there in front of everyone, I couldn't say a word. It felt like the ground had disappeared and I was being sucked into this endless black hole.

I snapped back to the sound of my mother crying, "It should be me! My daughter is too young to have this happen to her."Strangely, I accepted the fact. I knew my past better than anyone did. I began having sex at about fourteen years old because I kept falling in love with everyone but me. The day was long. My family and friends came to visit and I told everyone that I was HIV positive. On November 26, I went home.

I have regained the use of my arms and legs. I was given anti-retro viral meds to take on January 7, 2007. I take them everyday but I live with the knowledge that I am alive.

I am currently enrolled in a GED program and hoping to live my dream as a hairstylist. I can't say who infected me, or who I infected, but I can say, "It wasn't worth it." Teenagers, take your time, get your education, and live out your dreams. Remember that love doesn't love anybody if you don't love yourself first.

Innocence Lost

I busted into tears, and my heart dropped through a hole that was endless. The ground had made way for my life to disappear right through my fingers. For three months, I refused to believe that the earth was shaking and the ground beneath me was definitely caving in.

I sat across the room looking at Ora's hazel eyes, caramel colored skin and her hair that was pulled back into a ball, as she attempted to offer words of comfort to her friend. I knew there was something to be told about her life. She seemed sure that everything was going to be all right despite her current situation. Ora casually enjoyed her cookies and cheeses as she listened to others discuss issues around the wellness university. I wanted to know her story. After talking with her for over three hours, the losses and gains in her life weaved a tale that is so uncommon yet it has become quite common.

Ora told her story at times like a person outside of herself. At other times, she was so caught up in the memory that tears replaced her words. We began talking around 9:00 p.m. one night and the conversation ended early the next morning. Ora's life story played out like this.

Ora asked me to hold the line for a minute while she got a glass of water. She returned to the phone as a twelve-year-old girl growing up in South Memphis. She told me that she, her brother, and mother shared the house of a man named Mr. Bill, an older gentleman. He was one of her mother's "friends." Being a friend of my mother, he decided one day to help himself to me. I fought him off and ran away to a friend's house.

My mother soon came to get me and questioned my actions. I told her that Mr. Bill had tried to force himself on me. Believing me, she asked Ms. Sticks, an old family friend, if I could stay with her for awhile. Two days later, sitting in my temporary bedroom, I heard that my mother was across the street at Jesse's house (another one of mother's friends). I rushed to the door, and was stopped dead in my tracks, feeling that I shouldn't go outside! I could see through the living room window that my mother was being carried out of a car and placed on the ground (she suffered with seizures). The ambulance was called, and by the time I had forced my way to the street, they were placing a sheet over her face.

Through her tears, Ora said, "My mother was dead." I was twelve years old. My grand-mother came to get me. After the funeral, my grandmother's house became my home. I told my grandmother about Mr. Bill. Life became different for me. I was forced to grow up fast. Before I could celebrate my thirteenth birthday, I would be pinned in the grips of my aunt's boyfriend.

While babysitting for Aunt Lynn, Whiskey made his way into town. He was an over-the-road truck driver and my aunt's boyfriend. Whiskey and my aunt were in the back room talking as I fell asleep on the couch. I was awakened by a male figure who forced me to lie on my stomach while he grabbed at my shorts. As he forced himself on me, his hand covered my mouth. While turning my head trying to free myself, I saw my aunt's shadow in the door across the room. I still wonder why she didn't try to stop him. She just walked away as if what was happening to me didn't matter. When I told her, she blamed me. My grandmother picked me up the next morning for school. I felt worthless, unwanted, and unloved. My thoughts were unfocused and I had no direction. I failed the seventh grade. My grandmother had instilled in me by now that a man only wants one thing, and then he will be gone. That ranged in my head, so I thought Whiskey was gone.

By my thirteenth birthday, I had learned to play the game. I had a neighborhood boyfriend but our relationship was just puppy love. He would visit me, then go right across the yard, and get with my friend, Ann. She had his baby and that was the end of us. Whiskey was still in the picture. I had to babysit my little cousins and Whiskey had to have me, so I charged him. Why not? If you can't beat um, join um. My price was whatever I said it was—$100, $150, $250. He paid, my aunt was at work, and the children were taken care of. We all benefited.

By fifteen, I had fallen in love with Darryl. We were a couple until I was seventeen, or until I discovered I was pregnant. He got caught up in a twenty-five dollar bet with his baby's momma and her friends. The deal was that she could take him from me. She did. He would not return my phone calls and everyone told me how they would see them walking and holding hands. Even my grandmother knew. This hurt me to my core. I just wanted to tell him that I was going to be his baby's momma, too.

That would change when my Aunt Ruth saw me. Aunt Ruth was cool before she got strung on heroin. She asked me if I was pregnant and insisted that I go to the doctor. She drove me to a clinic— not a doctor's office. She convinced me that I was not ready for a child and that my life would be better without one. I loved and believed Aunt Ruth. While on the exam table, I wanted so badly to scream, "Stop," and get up, but felt I had gone too far to turn around. I walked out of the clinic numb but aching. I told Daryl, when he called me two weeks later about the baby; rather, that the baby was no more. I was in the eleventh grade.

Darryl was gone and in came Ken. He was younger, and the kind who thought that it was fun getting it on with an older woman. The sex was okay, but our time together was very short. I loved and still wanted Darryl back. Darryl, the baby and Ken, became things in my past. I returned to my life of drugs. I had been introduced to drugs while living with and around my uncles who used and sold them. I began to sell and use myself. They first introduced me to marijuana when I was only thirteen. By fifteen, I had moved up to cocaine, and two years later, I was rocking "crack cocaine." They didn't give me the stuff. I stole most of it from them. I was still only smoking marijuana but had a group of friends who liked it all, even pills.

I was first introduced to pills by a stranger—a white man. One day while walking with my friends to school, he pulled up alongside us and asked if we wanted a ride. We thanked him and declined his offer. He then asked if we knew where he could find some drugs.

Me being the more mature one, said, "I don't know what you're talking about. You could be the police."

"I'm not the police," he said quickly, "and to prove it, take this."

The car came to a stop a few feet in front of us. He handed me twenty-five dollars and a bottle with some pills in it. Then he drove off. I stuffed the money in my pocket and the pills in my purse. Pills were easy to hide because the school knew of my childhood illness. Having pills in my possession was normal for me.

I had no idea what the pills were, but I knew someone who did. My friend, Steve, told me they were black willows and I could get about $2.00 to $3.75 each. He was my first buyer—ten for $30.00. This was working better than weed. This new white friend was a friend for about four months. I had it going on. My purse was the school's drug store. I had pink hearts, 50/50, black willow, yellow jackets, teasing blues, and Delilah. She was my favorite at $25.00 a pill. I made it my business to arrive at school by 7:30, and before the bell rung at 8:00, I was at least $200.00 richer.

Everyone knew I had the good stuff, but one day things got out of hand. A girl got sick at school and threw up in the bathroom. Not just any throw up; she threw up pills and all hell hit the fan. If placed under enough pressure, people will tell on their momma. She gave names and I was one of them. I was called to the guidance counselor's office and questioned about dealing drugs on school property. Of course, I denied everything. My property was searched, but no drugs were found on me. However, down deep in a secret compartment of my purse was all the evidence they needed to suspend me; or worse, have me arrested. I knew they were in there and I knew I needed to get rid of them. I got my chance when the counselor left me in her office alone. I quickly took the pills out of my purse and stuck them behind some books on the shelf. I still wonder today if she ever found the pills and if so, what she thought. Alone with about one-hundred other students, we were given a board suspension for seven days. Upon our return, we promised to stay away from each other during school hours. Sure, we could do that.

Between running away from home, having an abortion, two miscarriages, and selling drugs, I never lived the life of a child, and I missed that. Anyway, I was going into my senior year of high school when I met Red. Red and I knew each other from the neighborhood. I was staying with my father's mother now and I was ready to go. My Aunt Debbie had snapped after a trip with her Christian group, and there was no rest in the house. After six months, I moved in with Red and his grandparents. His grandmother was blind. Red and I had both lost our mothers at an early age. Red was a few years older than me. He worked for a piping company and gift-wrapping paper company part-time. I continued to go to school and went to the doctor to get fitted for an IUD.

I continued selling drugs, and made connections in other states. I traveled to California, Chicago, Florida, and Texas. I knew transporting drugs was dangerous but I had to do what I had to do. I never sold drugs out of Red's grandparents' house. I carried a beeper, met my folks, or I would visit my drug houses. Transporting drugs caused me to lose a very good friend. One trip changed everything. Traveling back from Texas, we were pulled over by state troopers. She was driving, and I was the drug dealer. My friend took the rap for me. She was given eight years for the crime of transporting drugs with intent to sell. I didn't forget her. I kept money on her books, but heroin became her new friend behind the bars. She was never the same.

I married Red two weeks before graduation. I missed my graduation because my husband was in an accident. This really disappointed my family. I was happy, and business was good, until one day my IUD had become dislodged. I had to have it removed. The next thing I knew, I became pregnant. I stopped using drugs and was on bed rest for seven months. My son was born January 1990. I had stopped selling and using drugs, but things were getting worse between Red and me. He was still using and I could not take it anymore. I moved out with an older man named Ed.

Ed was fifty-three and an alcoholic. Having sex with him was a chore. Sometimes it's up, but most of the time it's not—if you know what I mean. I still kept in contact with Red because he was my baby's father, and I cared about his grandparents. Red had an uncle who was not of the Christian belief. He didn't eat certain foods. I found out he was coming to visit his parents, so I went over to the house and prepared him a welcome home meal. I did it up wonderful with cabbage, a roast, and potatoes. However, something happened that night. Red's uncle shot and killed him. I found out the next day when my grandmother called to say that Red was dead. I could not believe it.

Now a widow, I became $10,000 richer because of his death. I was still his wife. I was doing drugs again so the money did not last long. Ed became sick and retired from his job. He started receiving disability and drew some of his retirement money. I smoked up another $10,000. Darryl came back into my life. He spent time with Ed, my son, and me. Darryl was a diabetic now and was receiving disability. Ed died and I ran into Zack, an old friend. He was a shade tree mechanic and he moved in with us. I suffered two miscarriages over a two-year period. My life was spinning out of control. I needed to change some things so I moved to the other side of town. I tried to begin a new life with my son.

I still smoked weed and drank. One day, Galloway, the finest black man I had ever seen, crossed my path. He was about six-foot-two and had a body of steel, but was recently out of jail for stealing. The boy was fine. We got together at a hotel. When I saw him naked, I had a change of mind. The boy was hung like a horse.

I asked him, "Where do you think you're going to put that?"

He laughed and said, "Baby, I know how to use this."

I didn't trust him. The first night was spent playing cards, smoking weed, and drinking. I gave in two weeks later.

After about six months of being with Galloway, he began coughing up blood. I insisted that he see a doctor, but he refused. Galloway was still up to his old tricks of stealing and did several tours in jail—anywhere from sixty days until November 29. I was the reason for one of those trips. Galloway stole my son's social security check, and I tried to chop his hand off with a knife. Being on parole, he was back in the slammer. He met some woman while behind prison walls and didn't return to my bed. He left town.

Here I was all alone but not for long. One day while sitting on my porch, looking down the street at the crack house, I saw this man or was it a woman? I don't know but "fine" described the walk and character. I knew the drug dealer so I asked him who that fine thang was that just left his house. He told me her name was DA. I didn't care. I had to meet her. On her next visit, he told her that I had asked about her. She stopped by my porch.

We chatted and she asked me for a ride to the store. Trying to play hard, I told her I needed some gas. I would have taken her anywhere. We spent the evening at the park with my son and a couple of my nieces and nephews. DA had a child when she was seventeen but had given the child to his father. I wanted to know everything about DA. All of my questions were answered when she kissed me. Two weeks later, she spent the night at my place. We talked, drank beer, smoked a little weed, kissed, and had the best sex I had ever had. I had found my new love.

DA kept her place and I kept mine. I was known in my neighborhood as the person who would help anyone. A friend asked if I would help a girl who had lost her apartment and needed a place to stay for awhile. I did. This was the worst. She was the most trifling female I had ever known, but the one who changed and saved my life. I was broke and needed some money bad. She said that I could donate blood and get $25.00. That was in November 1999. I gave the blood and went home $25.00 richer.

The new millennium was looking good. She was gone and DA and I were really kicking it now. On the morning of January 25, 2000, I received a certified letter from the blood bank. DA opened the letter. The letter clearly stated that I may have syphilis or AIDS, and I should see my doctor. I was shocked and began to panic. DA convinced me that everything would be fine. With all the people they saw at the blood bank it was probably just a mix-up. I wanted to be sure. We went to the health department. I requested an HIV test. I had to wait two weeks for the results. That was the longest two weeks of my life. The results were positive. I was infected with HIV.

This couldn't be happening to me. I had to visit my own doctor. Dr. Brown and I were cool and I was sure she would tell me that the test was wrong. I visited her office, and requested another test. That was in February. The results were the same. I was HIV positive.

I went back to the health department, and requested another test. Since I wanted this test before their suggested three-month waiting period, I was charged a fee. DA paid. Another two weeks of pure hell. DA was right there at the health department. I insisted that DA stay with me.

It was March 15, 2000; the counselor told me again that I had tested positive for HIV. I burst into tears, and my heart dropped through a hole that was endless. The ground made way for my life to disappear right through my fingers. I was thirty-three and dying. I would go back to my primary doctor—my friend. She would help me deal with this.

Back at home, I called Zack, Darryl, and Floyd. I told them they needed to be tested. I even told my son about my disease. He was ten years old now.

I had lived in my neighborhood for over seven years and one month into my diagnosis. While DA and I sat watching a movie, we heard this big bang in the living room. Rushing through the door were five men. One of them was asking why I had cursed his niece out. Confused and shocked, the fight was on. We threw chairs, lamps, canned goods, skillets, or whatever we could get our hands on to defend ourselves. I ended up at the hospital with a neck brace.

I could not make myself believe this was because of an issue with a girl. I knew the news regarding my disease was spreading.

DA and I moved back to South Memphis into my big momma's old house. DA was there for me, but I was having a hard time dealing with my diagnosis. Our relationship ended about one year later.

I was now on meds, and taking about twenty-two pills a day under the care of my primary doctor. It seemed like our doctor-friend relationship was gone. She was once very talkative and appeared interested in my life. Now she was just a person I saw once every month or two who asked very little about me, my life, or my child. I felt she had placed me in a "those people" category. Her support was gone. I needed someone to tell me everything would be all right.

I came across a flyer that read, "PINIC: Food and Fun for those HIV/AIDS infected and their family." I decided to attend. I met the friendliest nurse in the world. I told her my situation, and she suggested that I transfer my care to her clinic. I did. It was the best move of my life. I felt at home, and was surrounded by people who had the same issues and needs as I did. I even joined a support group. God knows, I needed some support. I met Johnny. He was infected, too. We became a couple. No, we did not always use condoms. Our relationship lasted about three years.

I began to spend evenings alone again, until the day my phone rang. It was my Aunt Lynn. She was crying. Whiskey had forced himself on her daughter. What was I supposed to do? I never thought I was Whiskey's first, and I knew I wouldn't be his last. She began to apologize for the way she treated me and not believing or protecting me. My mind went back in time. I wanted to tell her so badly about my life after what Whiskey did to me, but what would be the use? I had not seen or spent much time with my family over the years. They did not accept my relationship with DA. Aunt Lynn began to tell me about my cousin who had died of AIDS, and a cousin living with the virus. For some strange reason, this made me feel part of my family again. She wanted to see my son and me. She told me the family had been asking about us. I decided to visit them at my grandmother's (father's) house.

My son and I showed up and everyone appeared happy to see us. Everything changed when I needed to take my medicine. My grandmother insisted that I use a paper cup. This broke my heart all over again. We left, having had enough of their ignorance.

I am forty now, and I have a new friend. He is not infected, but he knows I am. I'm a grandmother of a beautiful little girl. She has never spent the night with me but I'm still hopeful. I have been off medicine for the past six months and doing fine according to my doctor. I get tired, weak, and exhausted at times, but I'm still here fighting with the seventeen people inside of me, she chuckles. We all have them; maybe not that many.

Ladies, let it go. It's in the past. There is nothing you can do to change what happened, or did not happen. Holding on to what you want does not mean you're getting what you need. We are all put on this earth for something, and I'm still in search of that something.

Lessons Late in Life

May 15, 1997

I cried in disbelief. This couldn't be happening to me. The hospital room went black. I felt nothing. The earth had just gobbled me up.

Karlin is not your everyday bubbly person. Some days she just wants to be around the crowd but not part of it. Her laugh is the sign that lets you know she is listening and wants to join you. When Karlin laughs, it is from somewhere deep within her soul. It is like a child being tickled, and it makes you laugh. Karlin has seen some tough days and hard times, but she still has a softness in her voice that makes you want to talk to her. I spoke with Karlin just to see what was behind those dark eyes and funny laugh. She told me her story with a sense of determination.

When I was in the twelfth grade, I had to go to the hospital because of my diabetes. I never graduated from high school. I was a homebody and never really connected with best friends or had any girlfriends. Being the only girl, I stayed close to my mother. I dated a little but nothing too serious. I had only two relationships with men from the time I was eighteen until I was thirty. One lasted four months and the other about one year. The reasons were not about sex. It was because the relationships weren't going anywhere. They couldn't keep jobs, so why should I waste my time? I lived with my mother until I was thirty years old, but that all changed when my aunt got sick.

Aunt Rose had a stroke. She was seventy years old, and had no children. I agreed to take care of her. She was no stranger; I had known her all my life. She lived in Mississippi. While living with her, I became friends with several of my other cousins. They were excited to have me around. We became very close and they wanted me to have some fun for a change.

They showed me how to dress a thirty-year-old body and how to style my hair. I must say the wrapping made the package look damn good. They introduced me to the club life, and they taught me how to smoke a little weed. I was having the time of my life. They would also have these house parties. That was how I met Jake. He was fine. After about two months, I was like putty in his hands. I liked Jake, but I've got to call him a one-night stand. After that one night of sex, I never saw him again. I would ask my cousin about him and nobody seemed to know where Jake had disappeared to. My aunt's recovery was going well, and I continued to stay with her.

I soon met Frank and within a couple of weeks, Jake was but a passing thought. Frank worked at a chemical plant. We soon moved in together. He became my new love. One day while visiting my cousins, this older lady asked me if I was pregnant. I said, "No!" You know it, like old folks can look at you and tell you when you're pregnant. Something about your eyes or your neck is jumping or something. She was right. I went to the doctor and he told me I was two months and counting. I told Frank, and he was happy. He wanted a child. I wondered if the child was Frank's or if it was Jake's. I had our son in June 1986. I was thirty-two years old.

Within a year, I was pregnant again. I lost the baby six months into the pregnancy, and had to spend a few days in the hospital. I was allowed to hold him and in his death, I could hear him crying.

That sound is still with me today. Imagine hearing your child cry and not being able to comfort him. The doctor discharged me from the hospital, and I went back home to Frank and our son.

A year later, I was pregnant again, but something happened during my seventh month. I was rushed to the hospital and an emergency C-section was done. The doctors told us if she lived through the night, all would be well. She died. I never held her. I knew the crying of my son and did not want to hear her cries. The hospital gave me a picture of her and they took care of her burial. There was no funeral.

The next year, I was pregnant again. This time I carried my daughter full-term. The doctors informed me at her birth that a blood vessel had burst in her eye but her vision would be fine. We stayed in the hospital five days.

I felt good coming home with our daughter, possibly because now Frank might stop hinting that our son wasn't his. We could be a family. I later learned as my daughter grew, that she was mentally challenged. Life was good for us. Although we moved every year or so back and forth across the state line, we were always close enough for Frank to drive to his job. Something happened on one of our stays across the line. I began to get these boils on my hip and side. I would go to the doctor, have them lanced, but they would return. One time they were so bad that I was admitted into the local hospital for three days. I recovered and went back home. My life was being with Frank and our children. I had not forgotten about my mother, and I would visit her every so often. After being diagnosed with diabetes, mother moved in with my cousin. They took good care of her and I would call almost everyday.

One day my mother stepped on a staple, which infected her foot. She had to be admitted into the hospital. It had poisoned her system, the doctors said. She was in the hospital for a month, suffered a massive heart attack, and died. I blamed myself. I thought if I would have been the one caring for her, the way she cared for me, none of this would have happened. Everyone tried to convince me that it was not my fault; it was God's will.

There were no more boils, but one day I just wasn't feeling good. I called and scheduled a doctor's appointment. Frank dropped me off on his way to work. I sat there in the waiting room anxious for the nurse to call my name. I desperately needed something to make me feel better. The nurse finally summoned me, and I noticed that I was the last patient of the morning. She weighed me, and then took my temperature. It was 107. This sent up a red flag. The doctor drove me to the hospital. I was admitted and collapsed right there on the bed.

When I regained consciousness, the doctor asked if he could run some blood work on me. One of the tests would be for HIV. I just wanted to feel better, so I agreed. I called Frank to let him know that I was in the hospital and that he would need to pick up the children.

The next time I saw my doctor was when he gave me the news.

"Karlin, you tested positive for HIV, but we're going to run another test."

I said nothing. The next test revealed the same results. I was HIV positive. It was May 15, 1997. I cried in disbelief. How could this be happening to me? The hospital room went black. I felt nothing. The earth had just gobbled me up.

I mumbled, "You must have my results mixed up with someone else."

He assured me that was not the case and began to explain my condition. He told me all my T-cells were basically gone, and that I would need medicine to rebuild them. I spent the next ten days in the hospital thinking and wondering what would happen to my children. Frank visited twice, since he had to work and care for our children. I was being discharged. Frank picked me up outside the hospital.

We drove to the pharmacy to pick up my prescription that the doctor had called in. I wanted so bad to break down and tell Frank that I was HIV positive, but now was not the time. I had to get my children and get home. I walked in the drug store and felt like everyone was watching me—as if they knew I was infected. I reached the pharmacy counter, and gave them my name. The pharmacist passed me my meds and told me to go to a church, and find a pastor to talk to. He told me I was going to need it. He was talking as if I should prepare for my last rights to be read. I was HIV positive, and I was going to die. I believed it, too. I did not go to any church. I just went home.

Everything appeared normal. The dishes were in the sink and the children were happy to see me. I had to tell Frank. We sat down on the couch and I told him I was HIV positive, and that he should be tested. He didn't believe me and refused to be tested. We lived life as if my diagnosis had been a bad dream. He refused to use protection and I didn't force him. I needed to know much about this virus, what it had done, and was doing in my body. I knew I couldn't find that kind of information in our small town so we moved to Memphis.

I found the help I needed at the Med-Plex. There were doctors who treated patients with my disease everyday. They also connected me with other agencies for service in the city. I began to feel I would live and not die. I had told none of my new friends outside of the clinic about my disease. I would hide my medicine in the drawer when they would visit my house. I thought if they knew about my disease, they would not be my friend.

My son would pick up my medicine every month and I would tell him, "Do not look in the bag. Just bring my medicine to me."

When I told this to my counselor, he laughed.

"Think about it," he said. "What if you were twelve and your mother told you not to look at something. What would you do?"

He helped me to understand and to tell my son.

I thought telling my son would make him run away or worse. After telling him with the help of my counselor, he gave me the biggest hug.

He said, "Momma, I will always love you no matter what."

I felt I could do this now. I've never told my daughter. I feel she just would not understand. She is dealing with a major ordeal in her own life.

At fourteen, she was raped and held captive by a neighborhood predator for over seven hours. It all happened one day when she was walking to school. He grabbed her and drove off. She was raped, tied up, and threatened. The school called me asking where she was because she was always at school. I told them I didn't know. I had sent her to school and she should be there. I became worried and went door to door in our neighborhood looking for her. No one had seen anything. I had my cousin take me to the school. When I got there, police cars were everywhere and my daughter was sitting in the principal's office. Her hair was a mess and her clothes were all dirty and torn. The police said they found her walking around the apartments next door and picked her up. She was questioned about what happened to her. One minute the man was tall and in her next statement, he was short. She was confused and very upset. We were taken to the hospital where she and her clothes were examined. She was given the morning-after pill and several other preventive shots. I was responsible for taking my little girl in for her HIV test. Her results were negative both times. She still has nightmares about that day and needs to sleep with me some nights. She is slowly adjusting; her grades have picked up and she is trying to live a normal life again.

Frank still refused to be tested, until the day he was admitted into the hospital because he wasn't feeling well. He was diagnosed with diabetes. After his discharge from the hospital, we went to the health department for his HIV test. The results were positive. He was asked to give the names of all his sex partners and I was the only name he gave. We never talked about it after that day.

The season changed to winter. Being laid off from his job during those months, Frank had to keep busy. One day while working in the yard, he stumped his toe and it just would not heal. A month later, he decided to go to the doctor. There was nothing they could do to save his toe and it was amputated. He would always pick at his foot. Due to an infection, they had to amputate his foot. Then within two months, they amputated his right leg below the knee. We were given an assistant who came to help once a week. Frank had to quit his job, and was eligible for disability assistance.

Frank would not sit still. He had to be doing something. While in the yard working on a lawn mower, he stumped his other foot and did not tell me. He could not accept being sick and would not take his medicine or eat properly to control his diabetes. One day his blood sugar dropped, and he passed out. I called the ambulance. They carried him out of the house in a sheet. He had lost so much weight by now. His brother and I followed him to the hospital in the car. After being discharged, the nurse came to visit. She noticed the sore on his left foot. He was admitted back into the hospital to have his other leg amputated. He lost his will to live.

I purchased burial insurance for both of us. I still have it today.

My life is not easy but I keep trying. Caring for a man who refused to move and a mentally challenged daughter makes my days long and discouraging, but I must go on. When your own brother covers the seat in his van, wipes it off when you get out, makes you eat off paper plates at family gatherings, and whispers behind your back that you've got that package, those are the days I just want to walk away from my life and start over, but I can't. I attend regular support groups and they have been a blessing to me.

Lessons learned late in life are still lessons learned. You have to keep it real, but most importantly, you have to keep it moving. Before your one - night stands or your long-term commitments begin, get tested. It is worth it. Your life is worth it.

From the Church and Back

August 3, 2003

The walls began to close in on me; the room was spinning and everything went black. My life is over. I can't go to college or do anything. I was going to die. I read the letter but missed the message.

I met Ashia about a year ago. She was this bright young lady who always wore hats. I began to call them her signature. Full of life, Ashia could hold her ground with the best of them. She appeared very wise for her age and the more time we spent together, I began to understand why. Ashia had lived a double life. She had everything a child could imagine, even love, but young adulthood would be spent searching for that love. Ashia began telling her story during the happier times.

My biological grandparents were deceased when my mother became pregnant with me. My mother worked for a very caring Christian lady who became my god-grandmother while still in my mother's womb. This allowed me to live a fairy tale life for five years. I recall some of those times because of the details, which were told to me, but some I remember very vividly. I remember the unconditional love that the bishop and his wife showed me. I remember spending weekends at their home, sleeping in my own room, and having the world as my candy store. I attended daycare at their church, and on weekends, I would spend time with the bishop and his wife.

My most memorable time as a child was my fourth birthday. The bishop's wife took me to a pony farm in Mississippi. I had never been on a pony before, and that memory is etched in my mind. It is funny when I look back now. I never really rode the pony except for about three minutes. What I remember most was my birthday cake and ice cream.

At the tender age of five, my split world was over. I was told by the bishop that I would not be spending as much time with them because I was about to start real school. He told me that I needed to be with my biological family more. They promised to always be there for me and assured me that they loved me. I always saw them at church on Sundays.

My life took a turn for the worse. I had been used to having my own room and now I had to share with my sister. I had all the attention and now I was fighting for the attention of my mother over the back of my siblings and her new man. I lived in a housing development where I was not allowed to go outside and play because of random shootings and drug dealers in the neighborhood. My time outside was under my mother's strict supervision. It was like having your favorite top ripped from your hand and tossed in a river.

I was not feeling positive about my sisters and brothers and they knew it. At the age of eight, my brother pushed me out of our two-story bedroom window. I suffered a broken arm, fractured both legs and collarbone. I was in the hospital for six weeks and confined to my bed for another six. When asked why he pushed me, my brother said he didn't and called me a spoiled rich girl. He said he was sick of me. Maybe I was still holding on to my times at the bishop's house.

While confined to my bed, the bishop and first lady came to visit me often. They helped me with my school work. I was finally out of the cast and learning to walk again. I went back to school and my mother decided to go back to school to complete her education as a way of getting us out of the projects.

By the time I reached my teenage years, my life had changed again. My mother landed a job with the Internal Revenue Service. We moved out of the neighborhood into a house. She worked this weird shift, having to be at work at 6:00 p.m. and returning home at 2:00 a.m. At that time, I was basically the only child at home. My brothers and sister were doing their own thing. I was left under the care of my stepfather. He was a truck driver. Sometimes he would be home when my mother left for work or would show up hours later, but would always call to check on me. I felt like the least-loved person in the world. My self-esteem was at its lowest point. I began to look for love in the streets and noticed boys. I spent less time with the bishop and his wife.

Concerned and suspicious, the bishop warned me to steer clear of boys who were not going anywhere, or who wanted nothing out of life. That information went in one ear and out the other. I was about to make my own decisions.

While riding my bike in the neighborhood, I made a new friend. A girl who lived around the corner from our house became my evening family. We became inseparable. Her older brother, Steve, began to show me attention. Being only fourteen, I lied and told him I was sixteen. He was twenty. He had a car and a job but above all things, he noticed me and complimented me often. We flirted for about a month before he asked me to sleep with him.

I asked, "Will you love me?"

Shocked, he asked, "Would you give it to me if I did?"

I said, "Yes."

His smile was my answer. I knew Steve would come to his parents' house so I made it my business everyday when my mother left for work and after my stepfather made his daily calls, to jump on my bike and head up the street. There he was turning the corner. He stopped and asked if I was ready.

I said, "Yes."

He wanted to know where I lived and if he could meet me at my place. I was not about to take the chance of getting caught by my stepfather so we went to a local motel.

I sat quietly in his car while he went inside, paid the clerk, and got our room key. We drove around to the room. I got out of the car, and felt very nervous. This would be my first time, but I wanted him to think I was really sixteen and had been in this situation before. After entering the room, we went straight to the sex—no talking or TV watching. I got up, took a shower, and then he took one. He gave me $75.00 and drove me back home. I made it in the house just as my stepfather was driving up.

I sat in my room all alone and felt like a whore who had just traded her body for money. Those feelings soon passed and I waited for my next rendezvous with Steve. My secret love affair with Steve lasted about two months. He would pick me up at our spot. We would go to the hotel every other day or so. Sex was traded for money. My money began to pile up. Being only fourteen, my mother became suspicious. I told her that the bishop had given it to me.

When I made it home after school the next day, my mother met me at the front door. She asked me again about the money. With anger in her voice, she said, "Don't lie about the bishop."

I broke down and told her my man had given it to me. She asked who he was and why he paid me money. I told her for sex. She burst into tears and promised me that I would be going to the clinic tomorrow for an exam and birth control pills. I stormed off down the hall to my room. I was burning inside with my own questions. Why had they left me home alone? Why did she have to work at night? Why was my stepfather always late coming home, and why didn't I feel the love that once made me feel safe and wanted? Why that, Momma? I didn't see Steve that evening.

My clinic appointment was at 3:30 p.m. the next day. I told the nurse I was sexually active and that my mother wanted me to take birth control pills. She examined me, talked about some things, and gave me my prescription. I walked back through the waiting room where my mother was sitting. We went to the drug store, picked up my pills, and headed home. My mother was off to work. She said she would call me when she went on break. I waited in the front yard for Steve. I had to be back home by 9:00 p.m., since that was the time of my mother's break. We left. When I made it back in the house, the phone was ringing. I quickly grabbed the receiver, out of breath, and said hello. My mother was on the other end questioning where I'd been.

"I was in the yard and didn't hear the phone right away," I said, in a breathless whisper.

I let her know it was not 9:00. We chatted a few minutes, and then I went into the kitchen to fix something to eat. I couldn't wait until tomorrow to see Steve. I did a little homework and was asleep before my stepfather made it home. I couldn't concentrate at school. I wanted so badly to see Steve. Before my mother could turn the corner for work, I was on the phone calling him.

A female voice said, "Hello." and I hung up quickly.

The phone rang right back, and a female voice asked, "Did someone just call here?"

I said, "Yes, I dialed the wrong number."

I jumped on my bike and headed to my friend's house. She was outside. Slinging my bike to the ground, I asked her if she knew who the woman was who answered Steve's phone.

She quickly said, "His wife."

I could have died.

"Why didn't you tell me he was married?"

"You didn't ask."

That statement ended our friendship. I jumped on my bike and headed home. Steve called two hours later. I answered the phone and a voice on the other end said, "Can I come and get you?"

I asked, "Why didn't you tell me you were married?"

"You didn't ask," he quickly replied.

It was like he and his sister had rehearsed this scheme.

He asked again, "Can I come and get you?"

I said, "No, and while you're spending your money on me, use it for your bills and wife."

I hung the phone up and never spoke to Steve again. Still in search of love, my next target was Leonard.

I was in the ninth grade and he was in the twelfth. Leonard was a known drug dealer and had his share of women. I didn't care. We hooked up. We would have sex right there at school—in the bathroom, the gym, behind the building, and anywhere we could steal a few minutes alone. It was rumored that the security cameras were just on the walls to scare us into doing the right thing. Nobody believed we were actually monitored. One day Leonard and I just had to get our freak on so we ducked into the girls' bathroom during class change. Little did we know we were on camera. Leonard was seen coming out of the girls' bathroom adjusting his clothes and I followed close behind. We were called to the office. Leonard was kicked out of school and I was placed on a three-day suspension. My mother was called to the school and I was responsible for telling her the reason for my suspension.

I refused to press charges against Leonard because he had not raped me. I had been willing. My mother was furious. Our drive home was a conversation of "whys." You know she called and told the bishop.

The bishop came over to the house to talk with me. I was sitting right in front of him but my mind was on the other side of town. I nodded at the right time and said "yeah" where I thought it really mattered. That was one rough Friday.

I went to church early Sunday morning, and only about five people were in the building. It was like the bishop's wife was waiting for my feet to hit the sanctuary.

Over the loud speaker, I heard, "Aisha, please come to my office."

I went up the side stairs and knocked on the First Lady's door.

A sweet gentle voice said, Come in."

She was sitting behind her desk. She slowly pushed her chair back and met me in the middle of the floor. It was absolutely glorious the way she embraced me then led me to a sofa in the corner of the room. Never raising her voice, she began to give me the facts of life. She even told me about HIV/AIDS.

"Baby, you can get his disease and not be able to get rid of it."

She warned me to be careful and to use a condom if I just had to have sex. I was shocked at that kind of language coming from her. I promised I would.

Kissing me on my cheek, she said, "I'll see you in the sanctuary. I love you, Aisha," she said, as I closed the door behind me.

Sunday service was great and I was going to do better. I put off dating for awhile. When I entered the eleventh grade, I decided to take Vo-tech classes. That was when I met Michael. I was officially allowed to date now but not wanting to rush into anything, I decided to have Michael checked out by my parents. I invited him over to the house. My mother made nicety with him, but my stepfather took him in the back room. They needed to have their man-to-man talk, I guess. They both came out smiling after about thirty minutes, so I considered him a great choice. Michael's sister and I were friends. We took some classes together. We dated about six months before we had sex. I remembered what First Lady told me so we used condoms sometimes. I felt my life was back on track. My mother's work schedule changed and we were spending more time together.

Now a senior, Michael and I were still kicking it. I was in love. Just when I began to plan for my future with the love and support of my mother, she got sick. She needed to have surgery. After two weeks in the hospital, my mother was back home and doing well.

Our senior class arranged to have a member of Life Blood talk to us about how important it was to donate blood. We were also told about their "Pint for Life" program. I wanted to do my part. It was the least I could do for someone who did it for my mother. I went to the blood bank and gave my "Pint for Life." Two weeks later, everything was about to change for me.

The church was having a big ball and I was going. I needed to pick up a few things so my mother grabbed the mail as we were leaving the house. She passed me a certified envelope from the blood bank as we drove down the street. I opened it, and began reading the letter out loud. As I read the letter, my mother's body went stiff behind the steering wheel. I continued reading and then placed the letter back in the envelope. When we returned home, I rushed to my room to get dressed because Bishop and First Lady were picking me up.

As I entered the living room all dolled up, my mother was sitting on the couch crying. I asked her what was wrong. She told me to just go and enjoy myself, and that we would talk when I got back. I said okay and rushed out of the house as I saw Bishop turning into our drive way.

The ball was absolutely wonderful. I received compliments all night long, and everyone loved my dress. The night ended too soon, and it was time to go home.

Bishop dropped me off in the driveway. I told him good-bye and thanked him again for the dress. I rushed in the house to tell my mother about my evening. She and my stepfather were waiting for me in the living room. Tears covered both their faces. Before I could tell her about my evening, she asked me to have a seat. She was holding the letter I had read earlier.

"Ashia, you may have HIV and you need to see a doctor."

I said, "No, First Lady said you can't get rid of HIV."

I screamed, and ran out of the house. Anticipating my reaction, my mother had spoken with Bishop earlier. She had asked him to wait outside when he dropped me off. I ran right into his arms as soon as I opened our front door. We cried together right there on the steps. Bishop left for home but assured me he would talk with me tomorrow. The morning couldn't come soon enough.

Trying to hold back my tears, I sat on the exam table as the nurse drew my blood. She told me my results would be back in two weeks. Two weeks later, I went to the health department to get my results.

On the morning of August 3, 2003, the counselor called me in, and asked for my ID. She told me I was HIV positive.

I said, "Say that again. My god-grandmother told me you can't get rid of HIV."

The walls began to close in on me and everything went black. I felt like my life was over. I couldn't go to college or do anything. I was going to die. I was only eighteen years old. The counselor assured me that my life was not over and that I could do anything I wanted to do if I took care of myself. I left the office holding on that statement. I had one matter burning in my head. I had to get to Michael.

When my mother and I made it home, I had to see Michael. I knew in my heart that he had infected me. I had been tested before we started having sex and I was negative. I went next door to my neighbor's house and borrowed her handcuffs. I returned home, and asked my mother if she would drop me and Michael off at the movies. I called Michael on her cell phone from the car. I sat in the back seat.

We picked Michael up. I quickly placed one handcuff on his right wrist and one on my left. I told my mother to take us to the health department.

Shocked, she asked, "Why?"

I screamed, "Just drive!"

My mother dropped us off at the curb, and then went to park the car. I literally dragged Michael inside the clinic. Michael was given a number and asked to wait until it was called. Being handcuffed to Michael, I followed him into his interview. We entered the room and sat across from the counselor. He had a chart on his desk. He verified Michael by his ID and asked if he wanted me to stay. I raised our arms showing the handcuffs. Michael said it was okay. The gentleman asked Michael why he wanted to have an HIV test. Michael told him that I had insisted that he take the test. The counselor thumbed through the chart, raised his head, and told us that Michael had already tested positive for HIV. I could have killed Michael right there in the room. I unlocked his handcuff and walked out of the room. My mother was sitting in the waiting room. We made eye contact and she followed me out the door. I could not believe that my friend, Michael's sister, or his family, had never told me he was infected. I couldn't believe Michael never told me.

I pressed charges against Michael the next day.

Although a senior in high school, I didn't graduate due to one required credit—English. I could not stand to see Michael's sister everyday, and she and I took this class together. I began to spend more time with Bishop and First lady. They helped me to put my life back in perspective. I graduated the summer of 2004.

I still had dreams of being a chef but first I had to face this disease head on. I went back to the health department. That's where I met Shirley. She was a social worker and told me about the Med-Plex. It was a place where I could get the help I needed to manage my disease. She made me an appointment for 9:00 a.m. the next morning. I arrived at 8:50 a.m., and the waiting room was empty. I was called back at 9:00 as scheduled, and went through all my paperwork and more blood was drawn. My follow-up appointment would be two weeks later.

I was totally surprised as I exited through the waiting room. People were everywhere. I wondered who would recognize me and if all the people waiting were infected. I dropped my head and quickly exited through the door. I went back to see Shirley. I told her that this place was not for me and that I could not go back. We talked and she offered to take me to lunch. Over lunch, she told me about St. Jude, and that it may be a better fit. I was still a teen ager so they would accept me as a patient. She dropped me off at home and called me later that evening with my new appointment at St. Jude.

I would finally get my day in court to face Mr. Michael head on. The judge called our case to the front. Fighting back tears, I told how I had met Michael and that he never told me he was infected, and now my life was over. The room was quiet and everyone seemed to be focused on me and hung on my every word. The judge interrupted me a few times to clarify statements in my story. I told how his family knew and no one told me, or my family. It seemed like forever as I stood there trying to let everyone know that my dreams were shattered because of his selfish act of love. I walked out of that room feeling proud that maybe one less person would be spreading this disease. Bishop and my family were proud of me.

Michael was later sentenced to eighteen years in prison for attempted murder.

I had been accepted to a school in San Diego, California (Culinary Art Academy). I would be leaving in August. Bishop and First Lady paid for everything. I left all my worries and concerns at the Memphis International Airport. I was ready to try life again.

After adjusting to my new environment and school, I informed my advisor that I would have to travel back to Memphis for routine doctor appointments. I told him I had cancer. My next appointment was in October of that same year. As a student in the culinary program, I was allowed to work in the campus restaurant.

While at work, I was caught in a daze one day, just thinking about home, and how I was going to live with this disease.

I was startled by a voice, "Excuse me!"

I turned around and who did I see but Mo'Nique. Yes, the that Mo'Nique was standing less than two feet away from me.

"I'm sorry, mama, what can I do to help you?"

She asked, "What were you thinking about?"

I said, "You don't want to know."

She replied, "Yes, I do. That's why I asked."

I told her it was too much to talk about now. She said she had time and asked what time I got off work. I said two o'clock.

She said, "I'll be back at 2:00."

She ordered a cocktail and some fries. At about 1:30, Mo'Nique was sitting outside the restaurant waiting for me.

We went to Red Lobster to talk. I told her my life story and that I was infected with HIV. She gently rubbed my hand and said everything would be okay.

"You know, Magic Johnson has HIV, too."

We spent the rest of our time laughing and talking about brighter things.

Mo'Nique was sponsoring an upcoming pageant for full-figured women. She wanted me to participate. I told her I didn't have that kind of money. She told me I was pretty and she would sponsor everything if I'd just participate. I did. Bishop, First Lady, my mother, and stepfather were all in the audience. I felt like the most beautiful girl in the world. Life was looking up for me again. My life in California lasted only two years. I moved back home to Memphis in 2006.

That year would really test my strength and endurance. My next doctor's appointment made HIV more real to me. I was placed on medication to better control my disease—only two pills a day. I really needed some help now. I met Anna during one of my doctor visits. She invited me to a Feast for Friends dinner and suggested I bring a friend. This was a dinner for individuals who were HIV/AIDS infected or affected. I knew no one I wanted to attend with me, so I went alone.

Nervous and scared, I approached the building. The place was packed. I sat at a table in the corner and just watched all the people moving around me and I wondered if they were infected.

Three young ladies came over to my table and one of them whispered, "Are you HIV positive, too?"

We laughed and talked the rest of the evening away. I think they helped save my life. Tony came over and joined us as we began to clear our table. He thanked us for coming and invited me back. I felt I had made some new friends.

Bishop was sick now and I couldn't stand to see him suffer. We were supposed to take a cruise together this year for my birthday. Three months before my birthday, he died. Mo'Nique still keeps in touch, I'm living life to its fullest, and trying to improve my culinary skills. I'm dating again and my partner knows about my disease. He is not infected.

So to you, I say, take a look in the mirror. Do you really like what you see? If so, that's great. If not, start today. You are a designer's original and there is no one like you in this world. So he lied. You believed it. So what? He's gone. He was not worthy of you. Get up and move on. Be smart, not stupid. You will never find love if you're looking in all the wrong places.

Wrong Choices

February 28, 1998

I thought about my child but cried uncontrollably for myself. I felt like dust just blowing in the wind....

Vera is a mature lady who loves her hair braided. She always mixes in a little color to spice things up. She has now given her life to Christ and believes in forgiveness even if the pill is sometimes hard to swallow. As she moves into her more seasoned years of life, Vera has seen some rough times at the hand of others, but plenty from her own doing. She's getting her life together now and looks forward to the many years ahead. Her biggest desire in telling her story is to keep someone from suffering as she did in the past. Read on as Vera recaps the years of her life.

At the age of twelve, Vera saw her mother arrested and thrown in jail for over a year, all for the sake of a man. Living in public housing during those times, the rules were strictly enforced. The residence was for the woman and her children only. Vera insisted that her mother would have the children hide her lover's clothes when the welfare agency representative would make their unannounced house calls. This time they didn't move fast enough.

With my mother in jail, my sisters, brothers, and I went to live with our grandmother. I called her Big Momma. My oldest brother, who was nineteen, lived with Big Momma. She had raised him from a baby. Times were hard back then. I had to chop wood, carry water for the house and was taught to cook at an early age. Being short, my Big Momma would have me stand on an old log so that I could reach the stove top. In spite of my situation, I felt good about myself. I had long hair and a shapely body for my age. My oldest brother thought so, too. He placed a knife to my throat one night and dared me to scream as he forced himself on me. This went on for about a week, until one day I decided to tell one of my teachers. She called my grandmother to the school. Big Momma could not believe what I was saying but assured the teacher she would take care of it. I left school early with her.

When we made it home, my grandmother tied me to my bed post and beat me like a dog. She accused me of lying on my brother and making her shame known in the community. My brother denied everything when she told him what I had told the teacher. He would have his way with me for the rest of my time there. This was one of the worst years of my life.

My mother was finally out of jail. She came to Big Momma's house to get me and my sisters, but she left the boys until she could find a permanent place to stay. I told her what my brother did to me. She went back to Big Momma's house and tried to choke him to death until my grandfather pulled her up. I was treated like a queen by my mother for about ten days. I had all the attention any one person needed.

I woke up one morning and my name was everything but Vera. I became bitch, whore, motherfucker and worse. My mother had become this strange woman to me. I could do nothing to please her. This abuse went on for about two years, until she decided that I was the problem and needed to be seen by a professional. I was taken to see a psychiatrist.

The sessions were going great and I loved talking to the doctor. I was asked on one visit to fit the pieces of a puzzle together but became very frustrated when the pieces were not going together fast enough. I began to scratch my head, which messed up my freshly done hair. My mother would always dress me nice for each session. She thought this showed the doctor how much she cared for me. After one of the visits, my mother asked me if the doctor had molested me, while she brushed my hair back with her hand. I told her no. I was just scratching my head when the puzzle pieces would not come together. She insisted that I had been molested and told my counselor. We went to court and everything. I could not lie on my doctor. He had done nothing to me. He was the nicest man I had ever met. The case was thrown out of court. This made my mother very, very angry.

When we returned home, she beat me with an extension cord so bad that I had bruises and scars on every inch of my body. She said that we could have been rich if I would have lied and said that the doctor had molested me. My mother's drinking got worse. I would suffer two more years of her abuse.

All of the children were finally back together and that meant a bigger check from welfare for my mother and her drinking. Life in the house was hard for me. I became close to my youngest brother, and he shared my pain. He would always help me through my beating. One day I had a glimpse of hope. I had stayed home from school. My mother and I were having a good time together, but after about four beers everything changed. She grabbed me around my throat, and with a pair of scissors in her hand, threw me to the floor and began cutting my hair. My brother came home for lunch and pulled her off of me. I bit her hand and promised her if she ever touched me again, I would kill her. I ran into a room and locked the door.

My mother threw the few clothes I had into the front yard and told me to get out of her house. My brother gave me $10.00 and told me to leave before she killed me. I spent the night in the park. I was only fifteen.

The sun was coming up and I had nowhere to go. I prayed to God. Then out of nowhere this couple appeared. A lady got out of the car and came over to me. She asked me why I was sleeping in the park. I told her my mother had thrown me out. She and her husband took me home with them. I thanked God for my new family. She fixed me a hot meal. We sat at the table and talked for hours. Her husband said very little. She showed me to my room. I fell asleep feeling my life was good. I went to bed in what I thought was paradise and woke up in pure hell.

Morning came. I got up, used the bathroom, and headed for the kitchen. Kathy was at the sink and her husband was gone. She asked me to have a seat and then poured me a glass of juice. She sat next to me.

"You're going to need some money if you want to stay here," she said.

I had never had a job in my life. I guess the look on my face tickled her.

She laughed, rubbing my arm and said, "Don't worry. I'll show you."

She told me to go to my room and rest. She said she would be in later. Kathy invited two women over to the house and brought them to my room. They were lesbians. Kathy instructed me on what to do while she watched. I just could not get into it. The women soon left. She sat on the bed and said maybe shoplifting would be easier for me to learn. Kathy told me how to do it. She dressed me in one of her big coats, gave me a shopping bag, and dropped me off at Sears. All I had was a house key and $100.00 in my pocket. She told me that sometimes you have to buy something to get something, but be sure you get more than you spend. Kathy was headed to Three Sisters and Goldsmith's department stores.

It wasn't that bad. I came home with a few things, mostly jewelry. Kathy showed up a little later with mink coats and all kind of stuff. She gave me a mink coat. I was hooked.

My mother had put out a missing person's report on me according to my brother. I would see him every now and then in the streets. I even gave him a few dollars for helping me out in the past. Shoplifting was good but the money wasn't fast enough for me. Kathy showed me how to turn tricks for at least $100.00 at this motel. I got paid for sex. Other times, all I did was listen or and had the pleasure of releasing some of my anger by spanking men. They loved it. The money was good. I had made about $500.00 one day when Kathy wanted me to meet her at the nightclub.

We sat around the bar drinking and flirting with the men. I had to go to the bathroom and asked Kathy to watch my purse. When I returned, Kathy was gone and so was my purse. I asked the bartender if he knew where she went. Wiping the counter down in front of me, he said she left with some lady. I asked about my purse.

He said, "I guess she took it."

The place was about to close, so he offered me a ride home.

I didn't have my keys so I knocked on the door and windows while he waited in the driveway. The car was in the yard but all the lights were off. No one answered. I knocked for over fifteen minutes and yelled Kathy's name at the top of my lungs. She never answered. We left. I spent the night with the bartender. I was homeless again at seventeen.

I was still very upset the next morning. He tried to calm me and in his calming words, he told me how he had watched me over the months and thought I was fine. I wasn't really feeling him but at the time, I had nowhere else to go. Our relationship lasted about six months. I was still shoplifting and turning tricks. He acted as if love was the next word out of his mouth. I could not have that. Having access to his house and a few valuables, I needed to make my move. I had a friend who also did a little shoplifting so I asked him to help me stage a robbery. We stole his coin collection. We pawned it and got about $2,000. I gave my friend $500.00 then we parted ways. I was going to go back to the house and act shocked but I decided to keep moving. I never saw Kathy again.

I took my money and moved into a hotel until I ran across my girlfriend, Martha. I later moved in with her. Martha was still living with her mother and three-year-old child. I taught Martha the tricks of my trade. We would wait until everyone in the house was asleep, and then we would make our move on the night. I gave her one rule to live by—get your money before you lay down with any man. Living with Martha and her family was cool, but I soon got bored and had to move on. I ran across Gladys at the liquor store. I was now twenty years old. She was headed to a party at some of her white male friends' house and asked if I wanted to go. I told her I did since I wasn't doing anything. We got our liquor and walked down to the grocery store to get a soda. Gladys noticed this guy looking at me.

She said, "Ask him to buy you a soda."

"I don't know that man."

"Ask him anyway."

I asked and he bought me a six-pack. He asked where I lived. I told him here and there. Then he asked me for my number so he could call me sometime.

I quickly said, "I don't know you like that."

He said, "My name is Otis."

I gave him seven digits, not mine, and left. Gladys and I walked to the party.

I could hear the music through the door as Gladys rang the doorbell. A very nice looking man opened the door and invited us in. He wanted to know who I was. Gladys did all the talking. We were drinking, smoking weed, popped a few pills, and even did a little cocaine. I began to notice that the men were slowly passing out. At the right time, Gladys and I turned their pockets inside out, took their jewelry, and split. I never saw them or Gladys again.

Needing somewhere to lay my head for the night, I went back to the store to look for Otis. He was still at work and appeared happy to see me. I waited until he got off. We talked outside the store and I went home with him. Otis still lived with his mother. I never went back to Martha's for my stuff. I officially moved in with Otis. I continued doing my thing while Otis worked at the junk yard and grocery store. He became jealous and abusive. That's when I had to move on. I met John and we hooked up for awhile. A year later, I was back with Otis but kept John on the side.

We moved into our own apartment. After six months, Otis had a brother who went to church often, so he married us right there in our living room. We never bought a marriage license or anything. Still sleeping with John and Otis, I became pregnant. Otis had his suspicions about the pregnancy, but I convinced him that the baby was his. When my son was born, I knew it was John's child. Otis became more abusive. I went to the only place I could with a child. I went back to my mother's house.

We had little contact over the years but enough for her to see that I needed her help. She allowed us to stay with her. She made sure I applied for food stamps and welfare, so the money was good. I started seeing Leonard and Otis a little bit, too. Two years later, I was pregnant again. I quickly moved back with

Otis and convinced him again that the baby was his. When my daughter was born, I knew it was Leonard's. I didn't see Leonard much after the baby's birth, so I never told him. Otis and I did okay for awhile until John came back into the picture. Within three months of my daughter's birth, I was pregnant again. I had another son. I knew immediately that he was John's. My middle brother told Otis none of the children belonged to him. I knew in my heart why he did it. He held a grudge with me from childhood. When we were teenagers living at home, he caught a neighborhood boy and me having sex. He told me if I didn't give him some, too, he would tell momma. I didn't and he told. My mother beat me but I had gotten used to the beatings by then. I lived in pure hell with Otis for another six years.

One day, I had enough. I called my mother crying and she gave me a plan. She said I had to be ready in the morning at 6:00.

Otis left for work at 6:00 a.m. every morning. I had put sugar in the car tank, which would allow him to get to work, but the car would be dead after that. My mother and one of her male friends waited up the street in a truck until the coast was clear. We moved everything but his clothes, a chair, and a few dishes. My mother was carrying a gun just in case things got out of hand. I was ready to start my new life. My mother had found the kids and me an apartment on Springdale.

Life was good for about one month. I was dating a policeman from Arkansas. Apparently, Otis was casing the neighbor's house and saw the children playing outside. He showed up one night with his brother, drunk, and kicked my door in. My police friend was there and warned Otis to leave before things got further out of hand. I was on the phone calling the police.

Otis's brother dragged him to the car while he screamed, "I'll be back."

I told my police friend to go home to his wife and I moved the next day. I didn't move far—just on the opposite end of Springdale. My girlfriend from the apartment told me Otis came back looking for us.

I was in a house now, and it sat right next to an alley, which worked to my advantage. I was now seeing James. He was good to me and my kids. After about two months, he became boring, so I was on the prowl again. I met this married man. The alley was perfect for his entrance and exit. He and James would have scheduled times to come and visit me. My girlfriend, Debra, had moved in with me and my kids. One day, I got James and my married friend's schedules mixed up. They both showed up within fifteen minutes of each other. They wanted me to make a choice between the two of them.

I said, "I want both of ya," and walked out of the house. Debra was left there to entertain them. I called the house about fifteen minutes later. Debra said they were still there and that she had given them some Kool-aid. We laughed on the phone. I went back home about two hours later and they were both gone. I never saw them again. People came in and out of my life and it had gotten easy for me now. "Here today, gone tomorrow" became my motto.

I was tired of the house and my surroundings. After about one year, my kids and I moved in with my cousin. I put my stuff in storage and Debra went back home to her mother. My cousin loved to party and so did I. We would hang out at the neighborhood clubs and flirt with the men. One night I flirted with the right man. His name was Donald. He had a job, some money, and a car, but he lived with his mother. Donald was just what I needed. We moved into this rooming house together. The place became a bit crowded for five people, so we moved into a three-bedroom apartment at the Clementine apartment complex. We were one of their first tenants.

Donald got me hired where he worked, and we were happy. We got married two years later. He was a good husband and provider for me and my children. Four months after we were married, my sister asked if she could move in with us. She was tired of momma. We let her move in. I moved my boys to the living room, and she and her son slept in their room. I began to notice that she and Donald would always be off in the corner grinning, but I didn't think much about it. Then one night, after we returned home from a night of drinking and fun at the club, I wasn't as drunk as Donald thought. He told me he had to use the bathroom, which was right across the hall from our bedroom. I always kept the light on in there for the children. I never saw the light disappear from the door of the bathroom being closed so I got up to check on Donald.

He was not in the bathroom so I went down the hall. I heard this snickering coming from my sister's room. I opened the door. There he was kneeling at her bed, pulling her panties down and about to give her oral sex. She was acting drunk. I went back to my room and got my shotgun.

I never kept any bullets in the gun because of the children. I locked my hands around the barrel of the gun and tried to kill Donald with it. I hit him upside his head, back, legs, face and anywhere it landed. He ran outside and I was right behind him. My sister must have called the police. When they showed up, Donald had blood everywhere—even on me. They ordered me to put down my weapon. I did. I told them what had happened. They laughed and asked Donald if he wanted to press charges against me. He refused. They left and we went back into the house to get out of the neighbor's view.

I put my sister and her son in the streets. It was cold and rainy, but I did not care. My son begged me to let them come in the house. I did. We stayed up all night. When morning came, I told my sister she had to go.

"Call your mother, tell her what happened, and see if she will let you come back home."

She did but never told our mother what happened that night.

Things got better between Donald and me. We lived in Clementine for another five years, and then moved to Jackson Avenue. We paid $800.00 to move in and never paid any rent for three years. The man who rented us the house gave us a contact number that belonged to a McDonald's restaurant. He never came back to collect rent or called for us to mail it anywhere. We lived free, except for repairs to the house. We were doing well until one night. Donald said he was going to the store but the boys couldn't come with him. He left. I told Jr. to follow him.

Jr. returned home to report that Donald had gone to some woman's house. Donald did not come home that night. Donald and I had makeup sex the next day.

I had to go to the grocery store but in my rush, I forgot my wallet. I came back home to get it. I went to the bedroom for my wallet and someone knocked on the front door. Jr. answered.

"It's some woman," he yelled back at me in the bedroom.

Donald was sitting on the couch. As I entered the living room, I could see a female holding a leather coat in her hand. She wanted to return Donald's coat and asked if I was his sister.

I said, "No, I'm his wife," and slammed the door.

That was the straw that broke the camel's back. I had to put my plan into motion.

Donald and I had been talking about moving to Detroit, Michigan, so if I told people we were finally moving, they would believe it. I had to get some money. No one knew about the incident with Donald and me. I began to spread the word that we were moving and needed to sell all our stuff. My cousin bought everything (two TVs, air conditioner, bunk beds, dining room set, sofa, and chair) for $500.00. She gave me part cash and the remainder in food stamps. I turned around and sold my girlfriend the same TV for $75.00 in food stamps. I told her she could pick it up in two days. I sold my other girlfriend a TV and air-conditioner for $150.00. She gave me $150.00 in food stamps and I told her the same lie. My cousin and mother came to pick me and the kids up for our Greyhound ride that night, while Donald was at work. My cousin hauled her stuff away the next morning. I was finally free of Donald and the South. That was in 1986.

My sister picked us up at the bus station in downtown Detroit. We lived with her and her family. I was bored and spent my days sitting on the stoop just watching life and Kenny go past. Kenny was a neighborhood policeman. My sister insisted that he was interested in me by the way he patrolled our street more than usual. I wasn't interested until one day I overheard her husband ask when we were leaving. It had been a year and was time for us to go.

I found an apartment down the street from my sister.

Life was going well for my children and me until I met my new friends from Chrysler Motor Company. They introduced me to crack cocaine, new liquors, and plenty of parties and good times. I partied so much I lost my kids to the Department of Human Services. My neighbor reported me for neglect.

My girlfriend and I were coming home from one of our three-day binges when I saw the police and this white woman putting my kids in the back of a car. I kept going. My girlfriend said if I stopped, they would put me in jail. I met Rivers while my children were away. He was an older man, about seventy-five, and he fell in love with me. He loved me so much that he put me on his bank account. That was a mistake. I went to the bank and withdrew all of his money. He found out I had smoked it all up. My plan was to spend his upcoming retirement check, but he had my name removed. Enough of River. I moved on.

I met Bonnie at one of my crack parties and we became good friends. She helped me get my kids back. She knew how to work the system. I had to stay half-high for about three days, go before a judge, and say that I was getting my life together and I could get my kids back. The kids guaranteed me a check to buy crack. I got my kids back and I was at it again. My two youngest lived with me. My oldest son was now ready to be on his own.

I spent most of the money on drugs and bought some food. When my drugs were gone, I would trade the food for drugs. My son learned to steal to feed himself and his sister. My daughter soon became a child of the streets, using drugs, drinking and staying out all night. She was given some bad drugs, which messed up her mind. I was unwilling but mostly unable because of my own addiction to care for her. She went to live with her brother, and Jr. stayed with me.

My oldest son came to visit one day and found me half-high at the kitchen table. He told me his sister, my daughter, was HIV positive. I fell to the floor crying. He told me she was going to be okay. We talked awhile and then he left. I went on a high so deep that night, that I couldn't remember anything. I woke up on my living room floor the next morning.

I stopped running the street. I did all my drugs in my house. I would go out, buy my drugs, return home, and lock myself in my bedroom. I would become so high and paranoid that even a knock on the door would frighten me. This went on for over four years. I got tired of the life and decided I needed a change.

My friends gave me a smoking party one night, and I smoked nonstop. I got so high I didn't even feel high. I stumbled into the bathroom, and looked in the mirror. What I saw frightened me. I was a shell of the person I used to be. My eyes were bulging out of my head, my hair was a mess, and I weighed about eighty-five pounds. I prayed to God.

"If you show me a way out of this, I will never return."

I heard a voice that said, "Call your mother."

It was three o'clock in the morning. I called her later that day.

My mother was now active in church and wanted desperately to see me. I had promised so many times that I was coming home, and when she would send me the money, I would smoke it up. This time she bought me a Greyhound ticket that I could not cash in. I was finally headed home for real. It was 1997.

My mother picked me up in downtown Memphis. The 130-pound daughter she had put on Greyhound returned weighing only eighty-five pounds. I could see the shock on my mother's face when I waved from the other side of the bus station. We embraced, and on the way to the car, she told me I needed to eat more and go to church. I did both.

I finally got myself together and went to church with my mother. On our way to church, she told me that my life in Detroit needed to stay in Detroit. She told me that I didn't need to say anything to the folks at church. I agreed with her. Something happened that Sunday morning. I felt like the preacher was talking directly to me. I stood up and fainted. When I came to, I had to tell the congregation what I had been through to get here. My mother's face was full of rage as I glanced her way while I spoke. What could she do to me now? I was older and she was not going to whip me. I kept talking. When I finished, it was like a burden had been lifted off my shoulders. I cried all the way home.

Jr. soon left Detroit and moved closer to me.

Within a year, I had gained my weight back and mother took me to apply for disability and food stamps. I had hurt my back on a job years ago.

After visiting my case worker one day, I stopped at McDonald's on my way home. I met Lymond. He wanted my phone number so I gave him my mother's number. I did not have a phone in my room so I had to talk on the kitchen phone. After about two months, Lymond would come and pick me up. We would go to his place to have sex. He was extra sweet to me. He introduced me to two of his friends and we began to have orgies together, just the four of us. They took real good care of me. This made my mother jealous, seeing me come home with a fresh hairdo and new clothes. She wanted to know what I was doing. She became so jealous she took the phone out of the kitchen. I told Lymond what she had done so he bought me a cell phone and would pick me up at my sister's house. She lived around the corner. We had put the Leonard incident behind us.

This lasted a few months, until Lymond and his friends wanted to bring another female to the group. I was not going. I was not into women. This party was over. I soon met this guy who worked at the Pyramid. He was cool but he worked too much for me.

I had saved a little money, and had grown real tired of my mother's face in my business. I moved into my own place. I met Anthony. He soon moved in with me. Our sex was off the chain.

One day I woke up with this terrible discharge that had a very foul odor. I went to the health department for a check-up. While there, I also took an HIV test. They told me that my results would be back within two weeks. When I made it home, Anthony wanted to know about my appointment. I told him I had a bad yeast infection and that I also took an HIV test. He asked what I would do if I was HIV positive. I paid his question no attention.

On February 28, 1998, I went back to the health department for my appointment. The counselor called me back.

He said, "You are HIV positive."

I thought about my daughter, but began crying uncontrollably for myself. Oh, my God, I am going to die. I felt like dust blowing in the wind. The question Anthony asked me earlier flashed back in my mind. Venus came to get me. She was the clinic's social worker. She was so kind and patient with me. She took me to her office and then walked me over to The Med to see a doctor. After seeing the doctor, she took me to lunch, gave me her phone number, and then took me home.

I told Anthony about my diagnosis. He did not seem shocked and moved out that same day. I was alone again but this time HIV was with me.

Within a month of my diagnosis, I was placed on medication. I took two pills a day. My oldest son came to Memphis for a visit. I told him I was infected.

He said, "Momma, you will be okay. Look at your daughter. She is doing fine."

His words were kind but I lived in denial for two months. I would seldom leave my apartment. During one of my visits with my assigned social worker, she suggested I attend a support group. That turned out to be a good thing for me. I found out I was not the only one infected with this disease. I began to enjoy life again. I called some of my friends in Detroit and told them I was infected. I suggested they get tested.

My mother called to let me know she was in the hospital. I went to visit her. I called a couple of days later to check on her and somehow we got on the subject of HIV and AIDS. She said people with AIDS were nasty and no good. I don't know what made me tell my mother right there on the phone that I had AIDS, but I did it. She coughed for what seemed like forever. I asked if she was okay. She finally caught her breath and told me she was okay and she loved me regardless. My mother was released from the hospital and I went to stay with her while she recuperated.

She told me to bring my own blanket, pillow, and towels. I had to drink out of paper cups, eat with plastic forks and off of paper plates. I would wash my mother's dishes and I would see her rewash them with bleach. She would clean every surface I touched with Lysol or something. I felt my mother could take care of herself so I went back to my apartment. My mother made me feel worthless, but most of all, she made me angry. To prevent those feelings in the future, I very seldom visited my mother's house. I needed to start my own life again.

At one of my support group meetings, I met Fred. He was quite the charmer. He moved in with me, and before long, I had given him control of my money and my life. He did not have a job and was known to smoke crack. I took care of him. I would buy us clothes and he would take them and trade them for drugs. After his sweet words of nothing, I would always take him back. He knew just what to say. Before he left me for another woman, my credit was ruined. I was and am in debt up to my eyeballs with bank overdrafts, clothes someone else is wearing and a phone bill over $500.00, but I am slowly fighting my way back.

I am now involved in my church and very active in the ministry. All the men are gone and I have new friends and hobbies. I'm really doing well with my new life. I hope to one day marry and grow old with my husband, but until then, God is plenty for me.

Never place your happiness or life in the hands of anyone else. Been there, done that. Got the T-shirt, mug and picture frame. You must first love yourself before anyone can really love you. It is not about the people, places, and things. I was looking for it in all the wrong places and in the face of strangers.

Street Life

April, 2000

How could this be happening to me? I had my share of women but could only think of five names. My life was disappearing into this black hole as I tried to hold myself together.

Daren could be called your typical small city male. His mischievous grin hid his inner thoughts. It told you there was an answer to your question, but you must figure it out yourself. Daren had lived a fast life. He had more money than the average person his age but it quickly went through his hands. Daren stopped in the middle of cutting his mother's grass to talk with me.

Daren began by saying that he had grown up in South Memphis with his five sisters and three brothers. He grew up in what he felt was an average family.

My mother stayed at home and cared for the children while my father worked at the Army Depot and did a little race car driving on the side. He was a risk taker; he even sold a little marijuana on the side. I learned at an early age that you have to protect yourself and yours. Fighting was my biggest thing growing up. I had curly long hair, so the girls were crazy about me. This made their men jealous so I would get into a fight at least twice a week just because of the attention. I got used to it.

By the time I reached my mid-teen years, little girls at school were too childish. Women appealed more to my favor. My cousin introduced me to smoking and selling marijuana. I was making big money and loved it.

My father gave me a two-door Cadillac with a sunroof. I put the power package on it—a thousand-dollar paint job, whitewall tires and rims, cleaned up the crushed velvet seats and kept a tank full of gas. You can say I was a Mack Daddy.

I was eating at one of my favorite restaurants and saw this older lady across the room giving me the eye. I got her number and a couple of days later we hooked up at the Holiday Inn. I had another one hooked. She would buy me gifts and other women would buy me stuff and bring it to my mother's house.

My mother would always say, "Boy, you better quit what you're doing."

I never confessed to anything regardless of what she thought. I kept selling my dimes and quarters and sometimes thirties. After graduating from high school in 1984, I decided I was going to quit selling drugs and leave town but the money and my customers were so good. I just found it hard to let go. I stayed with the street games.

I needed a few new outfits one day, so I rode to the mall. I was a Marty and Goldsmith man when it came to clothes. I picked up a couple of silk sets and decided to lean on the corner with a couple of dudes before I went home. The police rolled up on us and ordered everyone against the wall. We were searched and I got my first offense. That was in 1985. I was taken downtown to the police station (201 Poplar). I used my one phone call to call my mother.

She said it again, "Boy, you better quit what you're doing."

I was given a six-month jail sentence. My mother kept money on my books and would visit me on weekends. I would call my girl collect about twice a week. I made sure she was not cheating on me. You know how we do it. I did the six months lying down (just chilling).

Out of jail, I had a cash flow problem. I quickly got myself back on my feet and things were going great. I got my own place and my girlfriend moved in with me. I was living the gangster life. I kept guns in the house but my favorite was a nine millimeter. I kept it on my side or in the back of my pants at all times. I hooked up with an old partner of mine. He became one of my sellers. I had to pistol whip him once about my money—you know, get them before they get you kind of deal. Everything was cool after that. He and I would make runs to Chicago or as far as LA. They were the kind of trips we turned into mini vacations. We stopped to enjoy the scenery before we headed back up the road. I had now made a name for myself and didn't need the middle man.

Needing to make some big money, I made a few phone calls and got the green light to pick up two kilos (bricks), locally. I got dressed and cruised to the location, picked up my stuff, paid the man. and headed home.

I had the sunroof back, thinking of how I would break the bricks up. Out of nowhere, I saw blue lights. Damn, I thought. I knew where I was going. I pulled over to the side of the street and got out of the car. The officer asked for my license and registration. I removed my license from my pocket and asked if I could get my registration from the glove compartment. They asked if they could search my car. What would be my excuse for saying no? I said yes, and then sat on the side of the road. That was in 1986. They popped the trunk and there in clear view were two gallon bags filled to the rim with white powder. I was handcuffed and placed in the back seat of the police car. My car was towed and I was headed to the police station again (201 Poplar). I used my one phone call to call my mother.

She said it again, "Boy, you better quit what you're doing."

My court day was set for one month later. My mother retained a lawyer for me to the tune of $1,500.00, and my bond was set at $75,000.00. I refused to pay the $250.00 bail. I was guilty and there was no way around it. I just wanted the lawyer to get a portion of whatever time I would be given on paper. This would cut my time behind bars short. I sat in jail knowing someone had set me up, but I'd probably never know who.

Dressed in orange, I had my day in court. Eight years was my sentence. I would do four lying down (behind bars) and four on paper (parole). My lawyer said that was the only deal he could cut. Two days later, I was on a bus ride to Northwest Penitentiary.

Dressed in my street clothes, I enjoyed the scenery during the ride to my new home for the next four years. There were about fifteen other men on the bus. Upon arrival, I was searched and given two pair of jeans and two blue shirts. This would be my only wardrobe. I was no longer Daren. I became Number 23. I was placed in a cell with Ronnie. He was cool, around my age, and was doing two years.

I never asked Ronnie about his charge and he never asked mine. We spent most of our time talking about girls—the ones we had and were going to get once we were out of this place. Ronnie was my new eyes and ears. He hipped me to what was going down on the grounds, who to steer clear of, and the known troublemakers. The routine was simple; up at 5:00 a.m. for breakfast, lunch was served at 11:00, and dinner at 3:00. These were the rules—everyday the same thing. I spent the time between meals in my cell or on the yard.

Yard time would always bring this strange tension. At a glance, you would think the guards with weapons who were posted all around had the control, but the control was on the yard itself. The place was run like directions on a compass. The north, south, east and west areas of the yard had their own guards among the inmates. You had to get in where you fit in. I spent my time on the yard lifting weights and watching my back. One day while lifting weights, I spotted a piece of metal about five inches long on the ground. I slipped it in my boot. I just might need it someday.

Back in my cell, I sharpened the metal and made a handle with some electric tape. I kept it under my mattress, but when I was out of the cell, it was always in my back pocket. Ronnie had warned me about a dude who bullied the yard. He called him a shit starter and a lifer. You know the kind, with nothing to lose. I became his target for some strange reason. He called me curly because of my hair.

In prison, someone is always going to try you. It is up to you to make a good impression the first time; this will set the tone for the rest of your stay. I was tried after only three weeks at Northwest. It happened so casually.

I was sitting in the rec-room just chatting with a few of the other men, when this dude, this lifer, bumped up against me. I pushed him and the fight was on. I grabbed my shank from my back pocket, stabbed him about four times in his stomach and chest, and walked away. As he lay their bleeding on the floor, everyone was ordered back in their cells and roll was called. No one saw or said anything. That is how it is done behind the walls. I had no other problems during my stay and laid down on the rest of my time.

I spent my time thinking about what I was going to do once I was free. I knew a life of drugs would not be the answer. I lived for my phone calls and visits from my mother. Four years passed. I walked out of Northwest Penitentiary.

Four years of my life were gone and four years remained on paper. The people I knew had moved on with their lives and the streets were different. I decided to go legal. I applied for a job with Southwest Services. This was a company that cleaned floors. I learned to wax as well as strip floors to restore their beauty. My assignment was at different local businesses and some university campuses. I was good at what I did. My work got me noticed by a gentleman at one of the universities who offered me a full-time job on his staff. I accepted.

Surrounded by all these college females made my work easy and I took advantage of all my opportunities. I dated what I liked at the moment. It didn't matter their race or religion. Everything was great. I had no ties and no commitments. Things changed when one female got a little too attached and reported me to my supervisor. I was fired for inappropriate behavior. Still needing to work, I answered an ad in the newspaper.

"Wanted: Individuals who have experience in sales, love to travel, and want to make money."

I got the job.

The job allowed me to travel to Chicago and Las Vegas, where I sold magazine ads to businesses and magazine subscriptions to families. The money was good. There was a group of about five of us. We lived in a local hotel, and we were picked up daily by the team leader in that city, and then dropped off to canvas different communities, door to door. The work was from 9:00 a.m. until 6:00 p.m. We would get picked up and driven back to the hotel and start over the next day. I would be in each city about two weeks. While on one of my stays in Chicago, I began to have these terrible headaches. I thought they were due to the weather, so I tried to control them by taken Tylenol. The headaches got so bad that I thought I would overdose on Tylenol. I was taking about ten pills a day with no relief. I needed to see a doctor.

I came home for awhile after my time in Chicago and decided to go to the Hope Health Center for my headaches—that was on April 12, 2000. While waiting to see the doctor, a young lady approached me. She asked if I wanted to take an HIV test. I knew very little about the disease so I decided to take the test. Within an hour, my life changed forever. The doctor examined me and gave me a prescription for my headaches. I was then seen by the lady who did my HIV test. She called me back to her office and told me I was HIV positive. It was as if someone had hit me with 210 volts of electricity. How could this be happening to me? I felt life disappearing out of me as I tried to hold myself together. I could hear the young lady asking me questions, but I just couldn't answer her.

I snapped back when she asked the names of my sex partners. Out of all the women I had slept with, I could only remember five names. As she wrote their names on her note pad, I wondered who had infected me. She encouraged me to see a doctor. Then she gave me a card as I walked out of her office.

The day was a blur. When I made it home, I told my mother and stepfather that I was HIV positive. My headache was gone, but I wished it would come back so that I could feel something. As I sat in my room that night, I stared at the card the lady had given me. It was for my doctor's appointment the next day. I never filled the prescription for my headaches.

My appointment was at 9:00 a.m. I arrived at the clinic at 8:45 and the lobby was packed. Waiting was the worse part. My time with the doctor and nurse were cool. They asked a bunch of questions. Few I could answer; other answers would be found in the blood they sucked from my veins.

In spite of all things, I am doing well now. I attend weekly support groups and detail cars on the side for extra money. I am once again banking on repeat customers but in a different way. I am in a relationship that has lasted almost three years. She is not infected but knows I am HIV positive. We use protection every time we have sex.

You can't hate the player; hate the game. Man down but refusing to stay there. Men: Check your radar; a pretty face and little waist could be carrying dynamite. Be careful and always use protection.

Until Later...

If not for the Grace and Mercy of God it could have been me. We have all witnessed the affects of HIV/AIDS on our nation and the world. This era in time will shape our history. HIV/AIDS will have an impact on who we are and where we're headed. I think it is still a message we need to hear and relevant even today. We have a lack of obligations and responsibility in today's world of sexuality. We have become an "anything-goes society."

If we believe the media, then everyone is promiscuous—jumping from one relationship to another without commitment or consequences. People are living together one minute and onto something new within months with little to no thought of the long-term effects. We view this type of behavior as part of our constitutional rights, but trust me, there is a price to be paid for such actions.

In the end, it really comes down to believing—our feelings are not facts. When the time comes that you enter into your first relationship, rekindle an old flame, or decide to try something or someone new, instead of relying on how you feel or what your bruised and battered heart tells you, get the facts. Take the test. Don't let your feelings override the truth.

The driving force behind what I've attempted to do in this book is to influence attitudes and enlighten. The risky behavior that perpetuates the HIV/AIDS crisis are particularly complicated because they involve our most personal feelings. They are often pre-disposed by deep-rooted social pressures and our upbringing. I strongly believe that in order to win the war against HIV/AIDS, we have to change. We must facilitate change and affect change. That includes changes in our beliefs, and changes in our attitudes, but mostly changes in our behavior. I mean no harm, but in the end…it's personal.

ABOUT THE AUTHOR

Mary S. Jones resides in Memphis, Tennessee. As an educator, trainer, and motivational speaker for over fifteen years, she has seen the face of HIV/AIDS change lives around the world. She believes that education is the key for change and that personal responsibility for self can stop the spread of this deadly disease. In the absence of a cure, and no sign of the disease slowing down, we must change our actions and begin to ask the important questions when it comes to relationships.

Life is too short and this virus is 100 percent preventable.

Mrs. Jones received a Bachelor of Education and Masters in Human Behavior and Management from the University of Memphis, and an MBA from the University of Phoenix.

Feel free to contact Mary S. Jones at www.marysjones.com

-Or-

5026 Arbor Lake Drive
Memphis, TN 38141
Phone: (901) 369-9880
E-mail: dafyr62@hotmail.com